# Behavior Problems in Children with Developmental and Learning Disabilities

**Robert J. Thompson, Jr., Ph.D.**
Fellow, International Academy for Research
    in Learning Disabilities
Department of Psychiatry
Duke University Medical Center

**International Academy for Research in Learning Disabilities
Monograph Series, Number 3**

**Ann Arbor      The University of Michigan Press**

Published in the United States of America by
The University of Michigan Press and simultaneously
in Rexdale, Canada, by John Wiley & Sons Canada, Limited
Manufactured in the United States of America

1989  1988  1987  1986    4  3  2  1


**Library of Congress Cataloging-in-Publication Data**

Thompson, Robert J. (Robert Joseph), 1945–
    Behavior problems in children with developmental
and learning disabilities.

    (International Academy for Research in Learning
Disabilities monograph series; no. 3)
    Summaries in French, German, and Spanish.
    Bibliography: p.
    Includes index.
    1. Developmentally disabled children—Mental
health.   2. Learning disabled children—Mental
health.   3. Chronically ill children—Mental
health.   4. Child psychiatry.   I. Title.   II. Series.
[DNLM:   1. Child Behavior Disorders—complications.
2. Child Development Disorders—complications.
3. Learning Disorders—complications. WS 350.6 T475b]
RJ507.D48T47      1986      618.92'89      86-6916
ISBN 0-472-08066-0 (pbk.)

*This series of monographs published under the sponsorship of the International Academy for Research in Learning Disabilities is dedicated to the recognition of Professor Alexander Romanovich Luria, Ph.D., of the Union of Soviet Socialist Republics, a world-class professional whose work underscores a major development in an understanding of the neurophysiological development of learning disabled children and adults.*

# Acknowledgments

I would like to acknowledge the contributions of John F. Curry, Ph.D., who has collaborated with me in the effort to delineate patterns of behavior problems in children. John has been a stimulating colleague and friend.

I would also like to acknowledge the contributions that Mrs. Brenda Maulden has made both to the preparation of this monograph and to the Academy.

# Contents

# Abstract

This monograph addresses the intersection of two childhood clinical problem areas that have suffered from conceptual and measurement ambiguities: learning disabilities and behavioral problems. The study of these two areas has been hampered by the lack of an empirically based system for delineating and classifying behavioral problems and by the reliance upon a main effect etiological model that viewed learning and behavioral problems as either organically or psychogenically based. However, progress is being made in delineating empirically based patterns of behavioral problems and in utilizing interactional models that seek to evaluate the role of biological, psychological, and situational variables in behavior and learning disorders.

Evidence from empirical studies is reviewed regarding frequency and pattern of behavioral problems in children in general and specifically in children with learning and developmental problems. One interactional model is presented, involving the delineation of behavior problems in children confronted with the task of coping with the chronic childhood condition of developmental and learning problems. The results of a series of research studies conducted through the Duke University Medical Center are also discussed.

Several main findings reflect our knowledge to date. There are many behavioral problems demonstrated in childhood but these can be reduced to a number of narrow-band syndromes and the ubiquitous broad-band syndromes of externalizing-conduct problems and internalizing-personality problems. These dimensions have been identified in many populations of normal children as well as children with clinical and educational problems. In terms of general group differences: children referred for care exhibit behavioral problems several times as severe or frequent as nonreferred children; those with developmental disabilities demonstrate more behavioral disturbance than normal children but less and different patterns than children referred for psychiatric care; and children with externalizing-conduct problems have poorer outcomes than those with internalizing-personality problems. However, it has also been learned that the frequency of behavioral problems in the normal population is high and that while there is some stability in behavioral dimensions over time, the consistency is generally insufficient to derive accurate prognostic statements for individuals.

Directions for the future are discussed in terms of both methodological and theoretical developments. While there have been methodological advances that enable empirical delineation of subgroups of children based on patterns of behavioral problems, there is a compelling need for theoretical advancement in terms of integration of findings and formulation of relationships among the various components and parameters, particularly in terms of etiology and outcome. Although most studies still employ a main-effect model, there is increasing recognition of the need to develop and utilize interactional models that seek to evaluate the role of biological, psychological, and situational factors in the etiology, intervention, and remediation of behavioral disorders. Subgroup formation based on a matrix of behavioral, social relationship, and cognitive dimensions offers the possibility for specificity of prevention and treatment intervention. The inclusion of a focus on the role of mediating variables, both those in the situation and in the individual, is one promising vehicle for enhancing our understanding of vulnerable and invulnerable children. An increased understanding of behavioral problems is presented as depending upon a new era of research studies that seek to be theoretical as well as empirical, that utilize interactional models, and that explore the role of potential mediating variables.

# Abstrakt

Diese Monographie beschäftigt sich mit dem Zusammentreffen zweier Problembereiche der Kindheit, deren begriffliche und experimentelle Behandlung bisher unbefriedigend blieb: Lernunvermögen und Verhaltensstörungen. Der Mangel an einem empirisch begründeten System zur Beschreibung und Klassifikation von Verhaltensstörungen und das Vertrauen auf ein Hauptwirkungs- und ätiologisches Modell, das Lern- und Verhaltensstörungen auf entweder organisch oder psychische Störungen zurückführt, behinderte das Studium dieser zwei Themen bisher stark. Beim Beschreibung von empirisch begründeten Mustern von Verhaltensstörungen und beim Verwenden von Interaktionsmodellen, die versuchen Rolle von biologischen, psychologischen und umweltbedingten Variabeln bei Lern- und Verhaltensstörungen festzustellen, zeigt sich nun jedoch eine fortschrittliche Entwicklung.

Beweisungsmaterial aus empirischen Studien wird überprüft hinsichtlich der Häufigkeit und der Muster von Verhaltensstörungen bei Kindern im Allgemein und spezifisch bei Kindern mit Lern- und Entwicklungsstörungen. Ein Interaktionsmodell wird präsentiert, bei dem die Beschreibung von Verhaltensstörungen bei Kindern, die während der ganzen Kindheit mit chronischen Entwicklungs- und Lernstörungen fertig werden mussten, vorgenommen wurde. Ebenfalls besprochen werden die Ergebnisse einer Reihe von Untersuchungen, die vom Duke University Medical Center durchgeführt wurden.

In mehreren Hauptbefunden spiegelt sich unser bisheriges Wissen. Eine Vielzahl von Verhaltensstörungen zeigt sich in der Kindheit. Diese können jedoch auf eine Anzahl von enggefassten

Syndromen und die allgegenwärtigen weitgefassten Syndrome
von externalisierenden Verhaltens- und internalisierenden Persönlichkeitsproblemen reduziert werden. Diese Dimensionen
wurden in vielen Gruppen normaler Kinder ebenso festgestellt,
wie bei Kindern mit klinischen Problemen und Erziehungs-
problemen. Hinsichtlich allgemeiner Gruppenunterschiede lässt
sich folgendes festhalten: Kinder, die zur Behandlung eingewiesen wurden, zeigen mehrfach stärkere und häufigere Verhaltensstörungen als Kinder, die nicht eingewiesen wurden.
Diejenigen Kinder mit Entwicklungsstörungen zeigen mehr Verhaltensstörungen als normale Kinder, jedoch weniger, und
andere Muster als Kinder, die zur psychiatrischen Behandlung
eingewiesen wurden; Kinder mit externalisierenden Verhaltens-
problemen haben schlechtere Ergebnisse als solche mit internalisierenden Persönlichkeitsproblemen. Es wurde jedoch auch festgestellt, dass die Häufigkeit von Verhaltensstörungen in der
normalen Gruppe hoch ist, und dass es schwierig ist, genaue
Prognosen für Individuen aufzustellen, da es zwar eine gewisse
Stabilität im Grad des Verhaltens über längere Zeit hinweg gibt,
die Beständigkeit im Allgemeinen jedoch ungenügend ist.

Richtlinien für die Zukunft werden hinsichtlich sowohl
methodologischer als auch theoretischer Entwicklungen besprochen. Während im Bereich der Methodenlehre Forschritte
gemacht wurden, die die empirische Beschreibung von von
Kinder-Untergruppen, basierend auf Verhaltensmustern zu-
lassen, besteht ein zwingendes Bedürfnis nach theoretischem
Forschritt hinsichtlich der Vereinheitlichung von Befunden und
der Erfassung der Beziehung der verschiedenen Komponenten
und Parameter zueinander, vorallem was die Ursachenforschung
und die Resultate betrifft. Obwohl die meisten Untersuchungen
noch ein Hauptwirkungsmodell verwenden, wächst die Erkennt-
nis, dass ein Bedürfnis nach Entwicklung und Verwendung von
Interaktionsmodellen besteht, die die Rolle von biologischen,
psychologischen und umweltbedingten Faktoren bei Ursachenforschung, Behandlung, und Heilung von Verhaltensstörungen
versuchen auszuwerten. Das Aufstellen von Untergruppen

basierend auf einer Matrize der verhaltensbestimmten sozialen Beziehung und kognitive Dimensionen ermöglichen spezifische Eingriffe zur Verhütung und Behandlung. Das Mitberücksichtigen der Rolle von vermittelnden Variablen, sowohl in der Umwelt als auch beim Individuum ist eine erfolgversprechende Methode, um unser Verständnis von empfindlichen und nicht empfindlichen Kindern zu steigern. Das Anwachsen unseres Verständnisses von Verhaltensstörungen hängt von diesem neuen Forschungsgebiet ab, das versucht sowohl theoretisch als auch empirisch zu sein, das Interaktionsmodelle verwendet und das die Rolle von möglichen vermittelnden Variablen untersucht.

# Résumé

Cette monographie traite de l'intersection de deux zones de problèmes cliniques de l'enfance, qui ont tous les deux souffert de l'ambiguïté de concept et de mesure: les défauts d'apprentissage et les troubles de comportement. L'étude de ces deux sujets a été freinée par le manque d'un système empirique pour délimiter et classer les troubles du comportement, et par l'emploi d'un modèle étiologique à effet principal traitant les problèmes d'apprentissage et de comportement comme d'origine soit organique soit psychogène. Cependant, des progrès sont en train d'être accomplis dans la délimitation de motifs empiriques de troubles du comportement, et dans l'emploi de modèles interactionnels cherchant à évaluer le rôle des variables biologiques, psychologiques et situationelles dans les désordres du comportement et de l'apprentissage.

Les observations issues d'études empiriques sont examinées, au regards de la fréquence et du motif des troubles du comportement, parmi les enfants en général et ceux avec des problèmes de développement et de l'apprentissage. Un modèle interactionel est proposé, mettant en oeuvre la délimitation des troubles du comportement chez les enfants confrontés avec la tâche de vivre avec la condition chronique enfantine de problèmes du développement et de l'apprentissage. Les résultats d'une série d'études conduite au sein de Duke University Medical Center sont également ment discutés.

Plusieurs découvertes principales reflètent nos connaissances à ce jour. Il existe beaucoup de troubles du comportement paraissant pendant l'enfance, mais ceux-ci peuvent être res-

treints à un nombre de syndromes à bande étroite, et aux omni-
présents syndromes à bande large d'externalisation par la conduite et d'intériorisation par la personnalité. Ces dimensions ont
été identifiés dans de nombreuses populations d'enfants normaux comme chez les enfants avec des problèmes cliniques ou
éducatifs. Pour ce qui est des différences générales de groupe: les
enfants apportés pour traitement montrent des troubles du comportement plusieurs fois plus importants ou fréquents que ceux
non apportés pour traitement; ceux avec des défauts du développement montrent un comportement plus troublé que les enfants
normaux, mais moins de motifs de troubles, et des motifs
différents de ceux des enfants apportés por soins psychiatriques.
Les enfants ayant un problème d'externalisation par la conduite
montrent une issue plus défavorable que ceux ayant un problème
d'intériorisation de la personalité. Cependant, on a aussi appris
que la fréquence des troubles du comportement dans la population normale est élevée, et que bien qu'il y ait une certaine
stabilité dans le temps dans les dimensions du comportement, la
persistance est en général suffisante pour tirer des affirmations
exactes de pronostic pour les individus.

Les directions pour l'avenir sont abordées en termes de
développements théoriques et méthodologiques. Bien que soient
survenues des avancées méthodologiques permettant la délimitation empirique de sous-groups d'enfants selon un motif de
troubles du comportement, il existe un besoin urgent d'avancées
théoriques quant à l'intégration des découvertes et la formulation des rapports entre composants et paramètres, particulière-
ment pour l'étiologie et l'issue. Bien que la plupart des issues
emploient un modèle à effet principal, il y a une reconnaissance
croissante du besoin de développer et d'utiliser des modèles
interactionnels cherchant à évaluer le rôle des facteurs biologiques, psychologiques et situationnels dans l'étiologie, l'intervention, et le remédiement aux désordres du comportement. La
formation de sous-groupes fondée sur une matrice de relations
sociales et de comportement, et de dimensions cognitives offre
une possibilité de spécificité pour la prévention et l'intervention

en vue du traitement. L'inclusion d'un accent sur le rôle des variables médiatrices, à la fois celles se rapportant à la situation et celles relatives à l'individu, est un véhicule prometteur pour affiner notre compréhension des enfants vulnérables et invulnérables. Nous présentons une compréhension améliorée des troubles du comportement comme dépendantes d'une nouvelle ère d'études cherchant à être théoriques autant qu'empiriques, utilisant des modèles interactionnels, et explorant le rôle des variables médiatrices.

# Sumario

El presente estudio examina la intersección de dos áreas de problemas clínicos relacionados con la niñez, en las cuales existe ambigüedad con respecto a la conceptualización y medición: los problemas de aprendizaje y los problemas conductuales. La investigación de estas dos áreas se ha visto impedida por la falta de un sistema con base empírica que permita definir y clasificar los problemas conductuales, y por la aplicación repetida de un modelo etiológico de efectos principales en el cual se establece que los problemas conductuales y de aprendizaje son de originen orgánico o psicogénico. Sin embargo, se están logrando avances en la definición de patrones empíricos de problemas conductuales, y en el uso de modelos de interacción que tienen como objeto evaluar los efectos de variables biológicas, psicológicas, y situacionales en los problemas conductuales y de aprendizaje.

Se revisa la evidencia obtenida en los estudios empíricos respecto a la frecuencia y los patrones de problemas conductuales de los niños en general, y específicamente en los niños con problemas de aprendizaje y desarrollo. Se presenta un modelo interaccional que incorpora la delineación de problemas conductuales en niños que enfrenten las dificultades de condiciones crónicas de problemas de desarrollo y aprendizaje durante la niñez. También se ponen a discusión los resultados de una serie de estudios de investigación llevados a cabo en el Duke University Medical Center.

Nuestro conocimiento hasta la fecha se refleja en varios resultados de investigación que tienen una importancia fundamental. Existen muchos problems conductuales que se manifiestan en la niñez, pero estos pueden ser condensados en términos de diversos síndromes de rango limitado y los ubicuos síndromes de rango amplio que abarcan problemas de externalización en la conducta y problemas de internalización en la personalidad. Estas dimensiones han sido identificadas en muchas poblaciones de niños normales así como también en niños con problemas clínicos y de aprendizaje. En términos de las diferencias globales entre estos dos grupos, se puede manifestar que: los niños que reciben tratamiento presentan problemas conductuales mucho más severos o más frecuentes que los niños normales; aquellos con problemas de desarrollo demuestran mayores disturbios de conducta que los niños normales, pero los disturbios son menores y tienen distintos patrones cuando se comparan con los niños que están bajo tratamiento psiquiátrico; y en los casos de niños con problemas de externalización en la conducta los resultados son menos alentadores que en casos de problemas de internalización en la personalidad. Sin embargo, se puede concluir que la frecuencia de problemas conductuales es alta en la población normal, y aunque existe alguna estabilidad de dimensiones de conducta en el largo plazo, generalmente no son lo suficientemente consistentes como para derivar pronósticos acertados al nivel individual.

Las direcciones futuras se ponen a discusión en términos de los avances metodológicos y teóricos. Aunque han habido avances metodológicos que permiten la delineación empírica de subgrupos de niños basados en patrones de problemas conductuales, existe una necesidad imprescindible para el desarrollo teórico en términos de la integración de conclusiones y la formulación de relaciones entre los diversos componentes a parámetros, especialmente en lo que se refiere a etiología y resultados. A pesar de que la mayoría de los estudios aun hacen uso de un modelo de efectos principales, se reconoce cada vez más la necesidad de desarrollar y utilizar modelos de interacción que intenan evaluar el rol de factores biológicas, psicológicos y situacionales en la etiología, intervención y cura de desórdenes conductuales. La formación de subgrupos basados en una matriz de dimensiones conductuales, sociales y cognitivas ofrece la posibilidad de especificidad en la prevención y el tratamiento. La inclusión de un énfasis en el rol de variables mediadoras, tanto en la situación como en el individuo, es un elemento prometedor tendiente a fortalecer nuestra comprensión de los niños vulnerables e invulnerables. Se concluye que los avances en nuestra comprensión acerca de los problemas conductuales dependerán de una nueva generación de estudios de investigación que deben ser tanto teóricos como empíricos, que utilicen modelos interaccionales, y que exploren en rol de variables mediadoras potenciales.

# CHAPTER 1
# Introduction

The purpose of this monograph is to describe the research schema that my colleagues and I have been utilizing over the past decade to investigate behavior problems and disorders in childhood and to discuss the findings in relation to children with learning disabilities. Thus, this monograph will address the intersection of two childhood clinical problem areas that have suffered from conceptual and measurement ambiguities: learning disabilities and behavior problems.

The emphasis of the research endeavors to be described here has been on resolving some of the ambiguities regarding behavior problems in children, rather than an emphasis on the conceptual, definitional, and measurement issues surrounding the nature of learning disabilities. The governing premise has been that efforts need to be directed toward developing a system for delineating behavior problems that can be used to assess the frequency and pattern of behavior disturbance across any number of meaningful subgroups of children, ranging from those at risk for developmental or learning problems or psychopathology to those with primary physical illnesses to those with frank psychopathology. The goal has been to form homogeneous subgroups of children, on the basis of commonality of behavioral disturbance, for whom specific treatment and prevention programs could subsequently be developed.

Although we are interested in the delineation of childhood behavior disorders in general, we have focused particularly on children, who, with their families, are confronted with the tasks of coping with chronic childhood illness or disorder. Chronic childhood disorders and illnesses such as cystic fibrosis, diabetes, and developmental and learning disabilities are considered as stressors that can tax the coping resources of children and families and that carry with them increased risk for psychosocial problems.

However, not all children with chronic illness or disorder develop behavioral disturbance. Some demonstrate remarkable resiliency and cope effectively with the stresses associated with their disorder. Increasing knowledge about the intrapersonal and environmental factors associated with vulnerable and invulnerable children may foster an increased understanding of the emergence of behavior problems and thereby facilitate the development of prevention programs.

Thus, embedding our study of behavior problems in the context of chronic childhood illness affords an opportunity to consider, both singly and in interaction, several dimensions. These include aspects of the stressor, the role of mediating intrapersonal and environmental factors, and the outcome response from good adjustment to behavior problems.

The major questions prompting our research to this stage have included:

- Can clinically meaningful patterns of children's behavior patterns be delineated?
- What are the frequencies and patterns of behavioral disturbances in children with chronic physical, developmental, or learning problems?
- Do the frequencies and/or patterns differ from those seen in children with primary psychogenic, psychiatric, or behavioral disturbances?
- If they do differ, in what ways do they differ and why?
- Will subgroup formation on the basis of homogeneity of behavior problem enable specific treatment and prevention programs to be developed and, thereby, improve outcome results?
- What are the interaction effects of behavior problem patterns and physical, developmental, or learning problems?

It needs to be stressed that the emphasis of this line of research is not upon a search for behavior problem specificity as a function of a particular chronic illness or disorder. There is likely to be as much variability in type and frequency of behavior problems within various diagnostic subgroupings of children, such as cystic fibrosis and cerebral palsy, as between diagnostic subgroupings. Rather, the search is for homogeneous behavior-problem patterns that are demonstrated, albeit with possible varying frequencies, across a number of subgroups of children. To date, the primary vehicle for our work has been children with the chronic condition of developmental disabilities. Our contributions with regard to children with the specific disorder of learning disability comes about by their inclusion in our developmentally disabled population.

The organization of this monograph reflects this research schema. Following this introductory chapter, the second chapter focuses upon the broad area of chronic childhood illness. Information regarding the prevalence of chronic illnesses and disorders in childhood is presented along with a consideration of the risk of associated psychosocial difficulties.

In the third chapter, developmental disability is considered as one type of chronic childhood disorder. The evolution of the concept of developmental disabilities—from its origins in the field of mental retardation, through the additive or umbrella phase, and up to the current functional perspective—is presented in some detail. This consideration is essential for gaining an adequate understanding of the array of problems and needs of this subgroup of chronically impaired children, as well as for appreciating the likelihood of a continued evolution of this concept as more is learned about the problems and needs of the developmentally disabled at various points in their life spans.

The fourth chapter contains an extensive consideration of behavior problems in children revealed through empirical studies reported during the last five to ten years—primarily those involving analysis of parent- or teacher-completed inventories of child problems and competencies, and, to a lesser extent, peer

ratings of social skills. Even within this restricted time frame, the
volume of research is extensive. The studies reported are representative but certainly not all-inclusive of this research literature. There is a focus upon findings with various normal and
referred subgroups pertinent to the issues of behavior problems
in developmentally and learning disabled children. Specifically,
the issues and findings regarding the range, frequency, and persistence of behavior problems in preschool and normal populations are explored. Particular attention is focused upon the stability of behavior across age ranges and situations and the resulting implications for: identification of children at risk for behavior
problems; the likelihood of effective intervention for identified
problems; and the persistence of childhood behavior problems
and psychopathology into adulthood. An effort is made to inte-
grate the findings regarding the social relationships of children
with behavior problems to provide a more comprehensive matrix
for risk identification and specificity of intervention.

The fifth chapter presents a consideration of behavior problems in children with learning problems. There is a review of
conceptualizations ranging from those that view learning problems as psychogenic, through an either/or approach, to an inte-
grative model of secondary emotional problems associated with
primary deficits. While it is argued that a range of behavior
problem outcomes can be associated with learning disabilities,
the conceptual basis for the postulated link between learning
problems and juvenile delinquency is considered. The integration of findings from several lines of research suggests the potential for subgroup formation among children with learning
disabilities on the basis of behavioral, social, and cognitive dimensions considered jointly.

The sixth chapter presents a synopsis of our studies at Duke
University Medical Center with children with developmental
and learning disabilities, children referred to a child psychiatry
clinic, and children with chronic illnesses. The seventh chapter
concludes the monograph with a consideration of the implications of the findings for clinical and research endeavors.

CHAPTER 2
# Chronic Illness in Children

Many of the once lethal diseases of childhood have now become chronic conditions. Advances in health care science and practice that are reflected in improved early diagnosis and treatment have increased the life span for many children who previously might have died in infancy or early childhood. As a consequence, both children and their families are in increasing numbers confronted with the task of coping with chronic illness over a substantial period of their respective life spans. (Thompson 1981, 1985).

American and British surveys report that 7 percent to 10 percent of children have chronic illnesses of primary physical origins (Mattsson 1972). Various estimates suggest that the total cumulative percentage of chronic physical disorders in children under eighteen is between 10 percent and 20 percent, if those with mental subnormality, emotional illness, and specific learning disabilities are excluded (Pless and Satterwhite 1975). If visual and hearing impairments, mental retardation, and speech, learning, and behavioral disorders are included, the estimated prevalence is 30 percent to 40 percent of children up to age eighteen who suffer from one or more long-term disorders (Mattsson 1972). Results from three large epidemiological surveys indicate that the leading cause of illness was asthma, followed by other allergic disorders, and then by the sensory and nervous system disorders of epilepsy and cerebral palsy (Pless and Roghmann 1971). Results from two epidemiological surveys indicate that one-third or more of the chronic illnesses of childhood are likely to be permanent (Pless and Roghmann 1971).

Chronic illness can be a stressor, and there is a substantial body of research regarding the association of psychosocial difficulties with chronic illness. The extent to which chronically ill children are prone to secondary psychosocial and emotional sequelae has been extracted (Pless and Pinkerton 1975) from three epidemiological surveys: the National Survey of Child Health and Development (Pless and Douglas 1971); the Rochester Child Health Studies (Pless and Roghmann 1971; Pless, Roghmann, and Haggerty 1972); and the Isle of Wight Survey (Pless and Roghmann 1971).

Findings from these surveys revealed that chronically ill children had, in comparison with controls, higher frequencies of significant discrepancies between ability and achievement test scores, a higher rate of reading retardation, and a 10 percent to 15 percent higher rate of psychosocial maladjustment. The risk of behavioral pathology was roughly proportionate to the duration of the illness and, to a lesser degree, to its severity. Maladjustment was more frequent among children with permanent illnesses than among those with temporary illnesses (Pless and Roghmann 1971). The secondary consequences may be more disabling over time than the direct effects of the illness (Mattsson 1972).

Thus, chronic childhood illness is frequent, and it can be a stressor with which there is an increased risk for psychosocial problems. Developmental disorders constitute one type of chronic condition, and our understanding of these disorders has been gradually emerging.

# CHAPTER 3

# Developmental Disabilities

The starting point for the evolution of the concept of developmental disabilities can reasonably be attributed to the appointment of the President's Panel on Mental Retardation by John F. Kennedy on October 17, 1961 (Thompson 1982a; Thompson and O'Quinn 1979). The panel's mandate was to prepare a national plan to combat mental retardation, and its report was instrumental in launching major federal service and training programs through legislation enacted in 1963. The major piece of legislation enacted was Public Law 88-164, entitled the Mental Retardation Facilities and Community Mental Health Centers Construction Act of 1963.

The legislative process of continuing the 1963 legislation and broadening the scope of its coverage provided the catalyst for the evolution of the concept of handicapping developmental disabilities (Thompson and O'Quinn 1979). Many professionals and associations testified regarding this legislation. Several key points were made. First, many common needs of individuals were classified under different diagnostic labels. Second, many of the retarded were also suffering other handicaps. Third, individuals with multiple handicaps required attention to all their physical and mental problems. Fourth, many people whose diagnostic label was something other than mental retardation had needs and required services closely related to those of the mentally retarded.

Subsequent legislation incorporated these points and brought under one umbrella disabled persons with common needs but different diagnostic labels. Developmental disabilities were initially defined as disabilities attributable to mental retardation, cerebral palsy, epilepsy, or similar neurologic conditions. Subsequently, the definition was expanded to include autism and some specific learning disabilities. However, because considerable disagreement arose regarding the definition, a task force considered the matter in 1976–77 (Thompson and O'Quinn 1979). The task force clarified that the term *developmental disabilities* was not a catchall for an arbitrary collection of existing labels or conditions. "Rather, the 'developmental disabled' are a group of people experiencing a chronic disability which substantially limits their functioning in a variety of broad areas of major life activity central to independent living" (Thompson and O'Quinn 1979, 14). A functional definition that cut across specific categories or conditions emerged and became the legal federal definition in 1978: A developmental disability is a severe, chronic disability of a person that

1) is attributable to a mental or physical impairment or constellation of mental or physical impairments
2) is manifested before age twenty-two
3) is likely to continue indefinitely
4) results in substantial functional limitations in three or more of the following areas of major life activities:
   a. self-care
   b. receptive and expressive language
   c. learning
   d. mobility
   e. self-direction
   f. capacity for independent living or
   g. economic self-sufficiency and
5) reflects the need for a combination and sequence of special, interdisciplinary, or generic care, treatment, or other services which are
   a. of lifelong or extended duration
   b. individually planned and coordinated

(Thompson and O'Quinn 1979, 14)

The major changes over the existing definition involved the replacement of specific references to categories of disabling conditions, such as mental retardation and epilepsy, with an emphasis on substantial functional limitations attributable to mental and/or physical impairments.

Thus, from its beginnings in the realm of mental retardation, the concept of developmental disabilities has evolved through an additive categorical phase in which a number of specific diagnostic categories of disorders were encompassed under one umbrella to the current common-denominator focus.

It is likely that the evolution of the concept of developmental disabilities will continue based on the common dimensions of substantial functional limitations and need for services. A functional perspective should enable a more complete delineation of the array of problems and needs demonstrated by the developmentally disabled with which the individual and his or her families must cope.

However, there are few reports that foster this fuller appreciation by detailing the problems and needs of youngsters and families referred for suspected developmental delay and disorder. Several reports have focused on categories of disorders, such as mental retardation (Wortes and Wortes 1968), learning disorders (Coleman and Sandhu 1967; Kenny and Clemmens 1971), or types of handicapping conditions and their educational needs (Forness et al. 1980).

## Multidimensional Findings with Developmentally Disabled Children

The need for such a comprehensive study of the complete array of problems, findings, and recommendations was addressed in a study of the interdisciplinary evaluation of a sample of 301 children referred over a three-year period to the Duke University Developmental Evaluation Center (DEC) for assessment of suspected developmental disabilities (Thompson 1982b). Since it is important to gain an appreciation of the major population with whom we have been working, the findings from the study of this sample are considered in some detail.

The DEC is an outpatient clinic of the Department of Pediatrics of Duke University Medical Center. Patients up to twenty-one years of age with problems in more than one dimension of functioning—such as speech, neuromotor, learning, or intelligence—that necessitate an interdisciplinary evaluation are eligible for services. The interdisciplinary team has members from the disciplines of pediatrics, psychology, speech pathology, special education, and social work, with experts in neurology, psychiatry, audiology, and physical therapy available for consultation as needed. A problem-oriented approach to patient management and record keeping is utilized.

At intake a developmental history and a preliminary assessment of the child's intellectual, visual-motor, and academic functioning is obtained by one of the members of the interdisciplinary team. This initial data base is supplemented with reports from the school and health-care providers and is presented at a staff meeting at which it is the full team's responsibility to identify problems and ascertain what additional evaluations are needed. Any complaint or functional deficit that requires management or diagnostic workup is listed as a problem. The degree of abstraction or specificity of a problem varies from symptoms, such as language difficulties or headaches, to specific diagnoses, such as expressive language disorder or autism. Subsequent to the completion of all evaluations, the findings from the specific disciplinary evaluations are discussed at a second staffing at which the full team arrives at a formulation, treatment plan, and recommendations. Interpretive sessions follow in which team members discuss the findings, implications, and recommendations with the parents.

Several factors were recorded and analyzed, including the demographic characteristics, initial presenting problems, findings arranged according to dimension of functioning, and recommendations resulting from this functional, problem-oriented, interdisciplinary evaluation process. These elements will now be discussed in detail.

The total sample of 301 patients consisted of 209 (69.4 percent) males, 92 (30.6 percent) females, 193 (64.1 percent) whites, 106 (35.2 percent) blacks, and 2 (0.7 percent) of other races. Ages ranged from eight months to seventeen years, with 6 patients (2 percent) less than two years of age; 56 (18.6 percent) between two and five years old; 143 (47.5 percent) between five and nine years old; 78 (25.9 percent) between nine and thirteen years old; and 18 (6 percent) were thirteen years of age or older.

The Hollingshead Two Factor Index of Social Position was used as a measure of socioeconomic status (SES) and was obtainable on 277 of the 301 patients. This index is based on occupation and education levels of the head of the household and yields five categories of SES from high (I) to low (V). There were 20 patients (7.2 percent) in Class I, 22 (7.9 percent) in Class II, 43 (15.5 percent) in Class III, 114 (41.2 percent) in Class IV, and 78 (28.2 percent) in Class V. There was a significant difference in SES level as a function of race ($\chi^2 = 51.18$, df $= 4$, p $< .0001$). While 69.4 percent of the total sample fell in SES categories IV and V, only 61.4 percent of the white patients compared to 84.6 percent of the blacks fell in these categories.

The most frequent presenting problems identified, in terms of the percentage of cases seen, were poor school performance (57.8 percent), speech and language difficulties (51.8 percent), parental expectations and perceptions of the child that were discrepant from the child's functioning (50.8 percent), and behavioral management problems (25.9 percent).

In terms of findings, mental retardation and functioning in the borderline range of intelligence occurred in 21.9 percent and 24.9 percent of the cases, respectively. However, half of the children functioned in the average-or-above range of intelligence. For them the problem was not intellectual impairment but substantial difficulties in other dimensions. Other medical problems were present in 27.2 percent of the cases, and 3 percent of the children had an additional chronic physical illness. Speech and language difficulties were identified in 43.5 percent of the cases and hearing impairment in 6.3 percent of the sample.

Central processing difficulties were a frequent finding. Visual-motor integration, auditory processing, and visual processing difficulties were found in fifty-two (17.3 percent), thirty (10 percent), and twenty-two (7.3 percent) of the children, respectively. Disorders associated with cerebral dysfunction were diagnosed in twenty-five children (8.3 percent). Of these, eighteen (6 percent) were diagnosed as minimal brain dysfunction (MBD, hyperactive), and three (1 percent) as having the Gilles de la Tourette syndrome. Fifteen children (5 percent) were found to have a seizure disorder. Thought formulation difficulties, including perseveration, poor integration, and deficits in abstract thinking, were found in thirty-one children (10.3 percent).

Medical findings occurred in 27.2 percent of the children. Other chronic childhood illnesses, in addition to developmental problems, were found in ten children (3 percent). Of these illnesses, six were cardiac conditions, one was pulmonary, one was genitourinary, and two involved musculoskeletal systems. Allergies occurred in nine children (3 percent). Failure to thrive (FTT) and feeding problems were found in three children each (1 percent). Nine children (3 percent) were found to have specific syndromes, and of these there were two diagnoses of fetal alcohol syndrome (FAS) (0.6 percent) and one (0.3 percent) each of neurofibromatosis, Down's syndrome, inborn errors of metabolism, and neural tube defect.

Hearing impairments were found in 6.3 percent of the cases. Of these children, three (1 percent) each had uniconductive and unisensory neural hearing loss. Bilateral conductive loss was found in 1.7 percent of cases, bilateral sensory neural loss in 0.6 percent of cases, and bilateral mixed loss in 0.3 percent of cases. Hearing impairment not further specified was reported in 1.7 percent of cases.

Visual impairment was relatively infrequent in this sample, occurring in 5 percent of cases. Of these children, two (0.6 percent) had strabismus, eight (2.6 percent) had poor visual acuity, two (0.6 percent) were legally blind, and three (1 percent were not further specified.

Neuromotor findings occurred in 19.3 percent of cases. Fine-motor difficulties were demonstrated by eighteen children (6 percent), gross-motor difficulties by twenty children (6.6 percent), and six children (2 percent) had both. Another twenty-five children (8.3 percent) had neuromotor findings that were not further specified. The array of learning problems and needs identified in this sample was extensive. Specific learning disabilities occurred in 15.3 percent of the cases, but many youngsters had substantial learning problems that did not warrant the diagnosis of learning disability. Similarly, for a number of children, educational classes or programs already existed that were appropriate to the child's needs and such resources could be recommended. However, for a substantial number of children, the educational recommendations involved not placement in a special class but modification of the content, structure, or techniques utilized in the regular classroom.

The findings also suggested substantial parental difficulties in coping with the stresses associated with developmental disabilities. Parent-child interactions were frequently found to be conflictual and many parents (16 percent) did not have appropriate expectations regarding behavior or capabilities of their child. Furthermore, many parents (17.3 percent) were experiencing difficulties with managing their child's behavior.

An array of affective and behavioral problems in descriptive or functional terms as well as traditional mental health diagnoses were demonstrated in 247 cases (82.1 percent). The most frequent were poor self-concept and low self-esteem in 66 children (22 percent), parent-child interaction difficulties in 61 children (20.3 percent), and poor interpersonal relationships in 24 children (8 percent). Emotional difficulties were also frequent. Of this sample of 301 children, 17.9 percent were found to be sad or depressed, 13.6 percent to be overly aggressive or angry, 12.3 percent to be worried or anxious, 11 percent to be markedly fearful, and 11 percent to be demonstrating feelings of vulnerability. Other behavior problems were found, including: distractibility (8.6 percent), short attention span (8 percent), poor frustration tolerance (3.3 percent), enuresis (2.7 percent), and encopresis (1 percent). Specific traditional mental health diagnoses were relatively infrequent: adjustment reaction of childhood or adolescence (4.6 percent); borderline disorder (1.7 percent); and childhood psychosis and autism in one case (0.3 percent) each.

In all cases the findings from the interdisciplinary evaluations were discussed with the family and various recommendations were made. Educational recommendations were made in 85 percent of the cases. Recommendations for a specific placement in a learning disabilities resource class were made in 75 cases (24.9 percent), in a special education class for the mentally retarded in 28 cases (9.3 percent), and in a class for emotionally handicapped in 7 cases (2.3 percent). Early intervention programs such as Project Head Start and developmental day care were recommended in 36 cases (12 percent), and therapeutic preschool placement was recommended in 11 cases (3.6 percent). The most frequent educational recommendation, however, did not involve placement in a special program or class. It involved consultation with the teacher regarding programs and techniques, which occurred in 135 cases (44.8 percent).

Recommendations for counseling or therapy were made in 178 cases (59.1 percent). More specifically, psychotherapy for the child was recommended in 104 cases (34.6 percent) and for the parent(s) in 76 cases (25.3 percent). Behavior management counseling for the parents was recommended in 75 cases (24.9 percent). In addition, family therapy was recommended for 10 families (3 percent) and marital counseling in 8 cases (2.7 percent).

Recommendations of a medical nature most frequently involved referral for some other specific medical service, such as otolaryngology, a weight reduction program, or ophthalmology, among others. This occurred in ninety-eight cases (32.6 percent). Specific recommendations for drug therapy or medication occurred in fifteen cases (5 percent). Referral for dental services was made in thirteen cases (4.3 percent).

Speech and language therapy was recommended for ninety children (29.9 percent) and audiological services for twenty-five (8.3 percent). Physical therapy was recommended for six children (2 percent). Referrals for various Department of Social Services programs (such as protective and preventive services, aid for dependent children, etc.) were made for twenty-three cases (7.6 percent).

A primary contribution of this study is a view of developmental disabilities achieved with a functional problem-oriented, rather than a categorical, approach. The array of problems and needs demonstrated by children with developmental disabilities and their families is extensive. Reliance upon a system that reported only the frequency of specific diagnostic conditions would substantially underrepresent the difficulties presented by children with developmental disabilities and their families, and would result in a less than full appreciation of the needed remediative and supportive efforts. This is particularly true of the affective-behavioral problems area. While specific traditional mental health diagnoses only occurred in 6.9 percent of cases, 82.1 percent of cases were found to have some type of affective-behavioral problem.

The second contribution of this study lies in providing a detailed clinical data base of developmentally disabled children with which to investigate empirical approaches to delineation and classification of behavior-problem patterns. Thus, while the detailed clinical findings regarding behavior problems stemming from a problem-oriented approach are important, what is more important is to go beyond the level of knowledge to delineate subgroups on the basis of behavior problems and patterns for which a specific intervention and prevention approach could subsequently be devised.

CHAPTER 4

# Children's Behavior Problems

The study of behavior problems and psychopathology in children has been hampered by the absence of a taxonomic framework or classification system within which research findings could be integrated (Achenbach and Edelbrock 1978). In addition, there is a need for standardized, objective, and reliable methods of measuring children's behavior problems (Thompson, Curry, and Yancy 1979).

Efforts at early identification of, and intervention with, children demonstrating behavior disorders have been hampered by a lack of empirical information regarding the types of problem behaviors and the incidence, prevalence, and severity of these behaviors among normal children. Furthermore, empirical data has been lacking regarding the relationship of behavior problems during the preschool years and later behavior problems, adjustment difficulties, and psychopathology (Coleman, Wolkind, and Ashley 1977). Thus, there is a critical need for both the classification of preschool children's behavior problems and a distinction between problem behaviors likely to remit and those constituting behavior disorders that endure, that will not remit without intervention, and that are reliable predictors of later behavior problems (Crowther, Bond, and Rolf 1981).

Not only is there a need for a classification system and for methods of measuring children's behavior problems, but the need is specifically for empirical approaches to measurement and classification. Such approaches must be firmly grounded in empirical data and should be expected to be more objective, operationally defined, and quantifiable than the traditional systems that rely upon narrative descriptions formulated through committee consensus.

These needs have been well recognized for some time and there have been numerous efforts to derive behavior disorder syndromes from behavior problems reported by parents, teachers, and clinicians. One frequently used approach to measuring behavior problems has been the construction of children's behavior checklists that are usually completed by parents and/or teachers. The ratings are subsequently factor analyzed to yield narrow-band and broad-band behavior problem patterns or behavior disorder syndromes. It has consistently been demonstrated that parents' and teachers' ratings of child behaviors can discriminate between children referred for mental health services and nonreferred children or normal controls. Checklists have been shown to be sensitive to changes in behavior as a function of therapeutic intervention with child guidance clinic patients (Zold and Speer 1971) and with mentally retarded patients (Tavormina 1975). Furthermore, despite the diversity of checklists, methods, and samples used, reviews have indicated considerable convergence in the identification of narrow-band and broad-band syndromes (Achenbach and Edelbrock 1978; Dreger 1981).

In their review of empirically derived syndromes, Achenbach and Edelbrock (1978) identified substantial consistencies in both broad- and narrow-band syndromes or factors. Two broad-band syndromes are evident: Undercontrolled, characterized by aggressive, externalizing, acting-out, and conduct disorder behaviors; and Overcontrolled, characterized by inhibited, internalizing, shy-anxious, and personality disorder behaviors. There is persuasive evidence for the narrow bands of Aggressive, Delinquent, Hyperactive, and Schizoid syndromes and good evidence for the Anxious, Depressed, Social Withdrawal, and Somatic Complaints syndromes. Other less frequent narrow-band syndromes include Sexual Problems, Immature, Obsessive-Compulsive, Uncommunicative, and Sleep Problems. Test-retest reliabilities for ratings by parents and teachers were quite adequate for both narrow-band and broad-band syndromes.

Thus, progress has been made toward the development of

empirically based classification and measurement systems. The findings of consistent dimensions of children's functioning across many populations suggest that these dimensions are genuine and robust. However, the findings are also beginning to point out additional needs if these empirical approaches are to have utility for individual patients. First, information regarding the epidemiology of behavior problems in normal populations and the degree of stability across both time and situations is essential to establish appropriate criteria for pathological deviations and guidelines for intervention. Second, there is a need for increased differentiation of the samples studied (Curry and Thompson 1979). The previously identified broad- and narrow-band syndromes may mask behavior patterns specific to more homogeneous subgroups. Third, it is necessary to translate scores on identified syndromes into categories of individuals or profile types that characterize groups of disturbed children and relate these profile patterns to other demographic and outcome variables (Edelbrock and Achenbach 1980). Finally, there is a need to demonstrate that empirical approaches can enhance the identification of those situations in which intervention, both primary and secondary, is necessary and effective. Essentially, this is a matter of prediction. Because the evidence indicates that two-thirds of children with behavior problems get better with or without receiving treatment (Levitt 1957, 1971), the effectiveness of therapeutic intervention cannot be truly assessed until it is possible to identify a group that needs treatment in the sense that its members will not get better through the natural process of development.

There are several critical questions that need to be addressed in the process of establishing a behavioral-science knowledge base about children's behavior problems. What are the types and frequencies of behavior problems demonstrated in normal children? How do behavior problems change over time? What is the association between childhood behavior problems and later adult adjustment? What are the types and frequencies of behavior problems demonstrated by subgroups of children?

In the following section, the research findings relative to these questions are reviewed. First, frequently utilized behavior-problem measures will be described. Then the evidence regarding the prevalence of behavior problems in the normal population, the stability of behavior problems over time, and the association of childhood behavior problems and adult adjustment are reviewed. Then, the social relationships of children with behavior problems are considered.

## Behavior Problem Measures

The number of instruments that have been developed to identify children's behavior problems is quite large (Thompson 1984). Several have been used most frequently and warrant the following detailed presentation.

### The Child Behavior Check List (CBCL) and Child Behavior Profile

These instruments have been developed by Achenbach (1966, 1978, 1979) and refined by Achenbach and Edelbrock (1978, 1979, 1981). The CBCL consists of 20 social competence items and 118 behavior problem items that parents indicated as "very true," "often true," or "sometimes true" of their child during the previous twelve months.

Factor analysis has yielded a number of broad-band and narrow-band factors specific to boys and to girls aged six to eleven and twelve to sixteen that has resulted in four editions of the Behavior Problem Profile. However, the two broad-band syndromes—Internalizing and Externalizing—and three narrow-band syndromes—Somatic Complaints, Delinquent, and Aggressive—are present in both age and sex groups. In addition, syndromes that featured withdrawn, schizoid, hyperactive, and obsessive behavior are found in all groups, but these dimensions differed somewhat as a function of particular age and sex groups. One-week test-retest correlations have been shown to average

.87, and interparent correlations averaged .67 (Achenbach and Edelbrock 1979). Intraclass correlations in the .90s for inter-parent agreement, one-week test-retest reliability, and inter-interviewer reliability have been reported more recently (Achenbach and Edelbrock 1981).

Substantial differences between normal children and clinical samples obtained from mental health clinics have been found on all scales. In terms of total number of behavior problems, clinical subjects obtained scores more than three times as large as normal subjects (Achenbach and Edelbrock 1979). In another study the prevalence of each of the 118 behavior problem items and 20 social competence items were determined in a study of thirteen hundred children referred for outpatient mental health services and thirteen hundred randomly selected nonreferred children (Achenbach and Edelbrock 1981). Multiple regression analyses were used to assess the independent relation of SES, race, and clinical status to each behavioral and social competence item within each age interval for each gender. Clinical status showed far more numerous and larger effects than race, SES, or age. Referred children had significantly higher scores on 116 of the 118 behavior problems. Although there was no overall tendency for more behavior problems or social competencies to be reported for gender, race, age, or SES level, there was a general tendency for behavior problems to decline somewhat with age and for parents of lower SES children to report more problems—particularly the undercontrolled-externalizing problems—and fewer competencies than parents of upper SES children. The behavior problems most strongly associated with clinical status across age and gender groups were unhappy, sad (or depressed), and poor schoolwork.

The Behavior Problem Checklist (BPC)

This instrument was developed by Peterson (1961) and revised by Quay and Peterson (1967). It consists of fifty-five items, each describing some child adjustment problem. Teachers or parents rate a child on each item on a three-point scale: not a problem, a mild problem, or a severe problem. Factor-analytic studies have yielded four primary dimensions: Conduct Problem (CP) consists of seventeen items that represent disruptiveness, aggression, and other behavior suggestive of acting out and poor discipline; Personality Problem (PP) consists of fourteen items that reflect nervousness, fearfulness, and lack of interpersonal competence; Inadequacy-Immaturity (II) consists of eight items reflecting functioning characteristics of immature children; Socialized Delinquency (SD) consists of six items associated with group rule-breaking.

In a review of a number of studies utilizing the BPC, Quay (1977) reports the findings of Speer (1971) and Zold and Speer (1971) stating that the dimensions of the BPC differentiated clinic children from nonclinic children and also reflected changes after therapy. Test-retest reliability is satisfactory. Evans (1975) obtained repeated ratings over a two-week interval that yielded correlations of .85 (CP), .74 (PP), .82 (II), and .82 (SD) for boys, and .91 (CP), .87 (PP), .93 (II), and .79 (SD) for girls from inner-city fourth grade classes. Victor and Halverson (1976) obtained stability coefficients over a two-year interval on first, second, and third graders of .57 (CP), .28 (PP), and .32 (II) for boys, and .74 (CP), .35 (PP), and .50 (II) for girls.

The BPC was revised again in 1979 to strengthen its psychometric properties by expanding its item pool. The Revised Behavior Problem Checklist (RBPC) has eighty-nine items that yield six scales or factors. The Conduct Disorder (CD) scale contains twenty-two items, the Socialized Aggression (SA) scale contains seventeen items, the Attention Problems-Immaturity (API) scale contains sixteen items, the Anxiety-Withdrawal (AW) scale contains eleven items, the Psychotic Behavior (PB) scale contains six items, and the Motor Excess (ME) scale contains five items (Quay 1983). Reliability and validity information on the revised scale is in the process of being generated.

## The Missouri Children's Behavior Checklist (MCBC)

This instrument was developed by Sines et al. (1969) and consists of seventy items describing the behavior of children. Parents are asked to indicate (yes-no) whether the child had demonstrated those behaviors during the previous six months. The items were drawn from several checklists and behavior descriptions existing in the literature to cover six dimensions of behavior: aggression, inhibition, activity level, sleep disturbance, somatization, and sociability. No items contribute to more than one dimension. The point-biserial correlation between each item and the total dimension score was at least .30, and the square of the point-biserial correlation was at least twice as large as the square of the correlation between that item and the total score on any of the other five factors.

Odd-even reliability for each dimension ranged from .67 for sociability to .86 for aggression (using the Spearman-Borwn correction), and the agreement between mothers' and fathers' ratings on individual items ranged from 53.2 percent to 93.6 percent, with an average agreement for all items included in each dimension from 68.9 percent to 93.2 percent (Sines et al. 1969). Thompson and McAdoo (1973) found correlations between mothers' and fathers' ratings of boys and girls to range from .20 on the somatization scale for girls to .78 on the aggression scale for girls, with an average correlation of .54. The clinical utility of the MCBC has been demonstrated in a series of studies that will be considered subsequently.

### Behavior Problems in Normal Children

A number of studies have endeavored to identify the dimensions of behavior exhibited by preschool children and elementary school children who have not been referred for behavioral, emotional, or educational problems. In particular, there has been interest in determining whether the dimensions evident in later childhood are also present in the preschool years. Richman,

Stevenson, and Graham (1975) used the Behaviour Screening Questionnaire that contains eleven problem-behavior items dealing with sleeping, eating, encopresis, attention seeking, dependency, relations with other children, activity, concentration, control, temper tantrums, mood, worries, and fears in an epidemiological study of behavior problems in 222 three-year-old children living in a north London borough. The findings suggested that approximately 7 percent of the three year olds had a moderate to severe behavior problem and 15 percent had mild behavior problems. There were no significant social class differences. Boys were found to be significantly more likely to be overactive, enuretic, and encopretic, and girls were more likely to be fearful.

Jenkins, Bax, and Hart (1980) described the prevalence and types of behavior problems found in a sample of 418 preschool children in north London. The mothers were interviewed at the time their children (who were six weeks to five years of age) were being seen for medical and developmental examinations. The findings indicated that the percentage of mothers worried about their child's behavior reached a peak of 23 percent for children three years of age and fell to 15 percent for children four and one-half years of age. The most common problems reported by the parents were: difficulty in management, 10 percent at three years of age and 5 percent at four and one-half years of age; child demanding too much attention, 14 percent at three years of age and 8 percent at four and one-half years of age; and temper tantrums, 22 percent at three years of age and 12 percent at four and one-half years of age. A relationship was found between developmental findings and behavior problems. Of the children with behavior problems, 35 percent had abnormal speech- and language-development compared to only 18 percent of the non-behavior-problem children.

Crowther, Bond, and Rolf (1981) used the Vermont Behavior Checklist to study the incidence, prevalence, and severity of externalizing (unsocialized-aggressive) and internalizing (socially withdrawn) behavior factors among two through five year olds attending day care. Teacher ratings were obtained on 558 children in the incidence sample and 709 in the prevalence sample. Relatively high incidence and prevalence rates of specific behavior problems were found, with the proportion of children exhibiting high severities of externalizing and internalizing behaviors varying considerably as a function of the age of the child and the behavior being rated. However, 20 percent or more of the males aged two through four and females aged two were rated as exhibiting high activity levels. Also, more than 20 percent of the two- to three-year-old males were rated as being inattentive and as demanding constant adult attention. Boys were rated as demonstrating greater frequencies of externalizing behaviors than girls, including destructive behaviors, refusing to do things when asked, having trouble coping with frustration, displaying high levels of activity, picking fights, and failing to pay attention. There were age trends for many of the externalizing and internalizing behaviors. The proportion of preschool children, both boys and girls, showing high severity of any given behavior tended to peak at two to three years of age and gradually decrease at four to five years of age. This "suggests that many symptomatic behaviors are age related and will show remission without intervention or treatment" (Crowther, Bond, and Rolf 1981, 39–40).

O'Donnell and Van Tuinan (1979) factor-analyzed a modified version of the BPC completed by nursery school teachers on 196 preschool children (mean age, 53.2 months). Results yielded six primary factors: conduct, personality, social withdrawal, attention seeking, hyperactivity, and distractibility. The pattern of correlations with congenital characteristics of sex, activity level, gross- and fine-motor incoordination, minor physical anomalies, and sociability indicated that the six primary factors could be collapsed into two broad factors—Conduct Problem and Personality Problems—and two narrow factors—Distractibility and Attention Seeking. The congenital characteristics contributed independent variance to the explanation of Conduct Problems (both sexes), Hyperactivity (boys), and Distractibility (boys). The principal sex difference that emerges is the consistent association of minor physical anomalies with the dimensions of Conduct Problem, Hyperactivity, and Distractibility for boys but not for girls.

In terms of the prognostic implications of early childhood symptomatology, Coleman, Wolkind, and Ashley (1977) report that for (fifty) boys there is no relationship, and only a slight one for (fifty) girls, between symptoms of disturbance at ages three and four as perceived by the mother and child's disturbance at age five as perceived by the teacher. There was some indication that overactivity for boys and separation difficulties for girls may be related to behavior in school.

In a study of the prevalence of behavior problems in children in kindergarten through second grade (five to eight year olds), Werry and Quay (1971) evaluated teacher ratings of 926 boys and 827 girls on the BPC. Many symptoms had high prevalence rates, such as restlessness in 49 percent, disruptiveness in 46 percent, and short attention span in 43 percent of the boys. Boys tended to have higher prevalence rates of acting-out or disruptive symptoms and total number of symptoms, while girls showed a slight excess of neurotic symptoms. There was also a tendency with both boys and girls for symptoms to decrease in prevalence between the ages of five and six and to increase slightly at age eight.

Normative data on the presence of behavior problems was provided by Stone (1981) in a study of approximately twenty-five thousand public elementary school children using a modified form of the BPC completed by teachers. The results showed that most children had very few problems and that very few children had a large number of problems. Over 36 percent had no Conduct Problem checked, and over 50 percent had two or fewer Conduct Problems checked. Over 28 percent had none, and over 50 percent had two or fewer Personality Problems checked. Only 5 percent had more than twenty-four Conduct Problems, and only 5 percent had more than eleven Personality Problems. Boys, regardless of age, had more Conduct Problems than girls, four to five on the average for boys versus two to three for girls. There was little difference between boys and girls on Personality Problems, both having between three and four on the average. Children in special classes for retardation and for emotional disorder had more behavior problems of both types than children in regular classes. Children at the lower levels of IQ also had more problems than those at the average-and-above IQ levels. These results differed from others reported in the literature in reflecting greater stability in number of problems across grade levels. Behavior problems were judged to be as prevalent and as severe in the primary grades as they were in the upper elementary grades.

McDermott (1980) reanalyzed the Bristol Social Adjustment Guides (BSAG) scores for all 2,527 five- to fifteen-year-old regular-school children in the standardization sample. Hierarchical cluster analysis yielded sixteen homogeneous syndromic profile types. Of the BSAG normative sample, 25 percent were defined as mildly to severely maladjusted. Of the maladjusted children, 60 percent manifested multiple syndrome maladjustment patterns, while 40 percent demonstrated only single syndrome patterns of maladjustment. Thus, the hypothesis of the existence of homogeneous multisyndromic profile groupings was supported. This is of importance because it is frequently the case in clinical situations that maladjusted children cannot be classified as evidencing one type of maladjustment but demonstrate elevations on more than one syndrome and differing degrees of maladjustment (McDermott 1980). Thus, the ability to generate homogeneous multisyndromic profile groupings through cluster analysis provides a means for translating a child's score on various dimensions into a meaningful behavior profile. Formation of homogeneous subgroups on the basis of behavior profiles could enable specification of etiological and prognostic parameters and increase our capabilities with respect to the essential task of identifying children needing treatment.

In summary, these studies of the prevalence of behavior problems in preschool children indicate that the frequencies are relatively high, peak around four years of age, and are higher for boys than girls. These studies have also demonstrated the existence of the two major behavioral factors in preschool children that have also been found consistently in empirical analyses of the problem behavior of older children. These are the externalizing or unsocialized aggressive behaviors and the internalizing or socially withdrawn behaviors.

## Stability and Change in Behavior Problems

Gersten and colleagues (Gersten et al. 1976; Gersten, Langner, and Simcha-Fagen 1979) have cogently pointed out that information regarding the stability and change of behavior problems is fundamental to the judgment of necessity for treatment and to the determination of the age at which prevention and intervention programs should be targeted for maximal benefit. The long-term significance of a behavior problem may vary as a function of the age at which it is demonstrated. A particular behavior problem could be normative at one age, and thus of little prognostic significance, but of considerable significance if demonstrated at another age.

Several studies have been geared to determining the change in various behavior problems and dimensions with age. Victor and Halverson (1976) used the BPC in a two-year follow-up study of a normal sample of children attending the third, fourth, and fifth grades. The results indicated stability for the dimensions of Distractibility (.54 males; .64 females) and Conduct Problems (.57 males; .74 females) for boys and girls, and for the Inadequacy-Immaturity dimensions (.50) for girls. Behavioral problems of young girls were more predictive of later achievement difficulties while behavior problems in boys were found to be more predictive of difficulties with peers and teachers.

Lindholm and Touliatos (1981) investigated the change in BPC factors in children from kindergarten through the eighth grade. Their findings indicated that the dimensions of Conduct Problem, Personality Problem, and Inadequacy-Immaturity (as well as psychotic signs) increased from kindergarten to third grade, declined from third grade to sixth grade, and leveled off at the sixth to the eighth grades. The dimension of Socialized Delinquency was found to increase up to the third grade and was likely to remain level through the eighth grade.

In a prospective longitudinal study, Kohn and colleagues (Kohn 1977; Kohn and Rosman 1972a, 1972b) provide information about the stability and change in behavior problems and competencies in children followed for five years. The subjects (Kohn 1977) consisted of a 20 percent random sample ($N = 1,232$) of all children three to five years of age attending ninety public day-care centers in New York City. These children were followed for five years until the oldest cohort completed the fourth grade. The bipolar behavioral syndromes consisting of Personality Problem Factor I — Interest-Participation versus Apathy-Withdrawal — and Conduct Problem Factor II — Cooperation-Compliance versus Anger-Defiance — differentiated children with known psychiatric disorders from normal children. At each age boys were rated more disturbed than girls on both Factor I and Factor II. There was also a marked increase in pathology, particularly with boys, as a function of increasing age. This was evident for boys on all measures and for girls on Apathy-Withdrawal. Teacher referral ratings rose for girls from 15 percent to 35 percent and for boys from 20 percent to 57 percent across the time period of this study. The median rate of persistence of disturbance of behavior problems from each age level to every other age level was 45 percent; thus, the rate of remission was 55 percent. For healthy functioning, persistence ranged from 38 percent to 49 percent; thus, the rate of deterioration was 51 percent to 62 percent. In general, stability of behavior decreased and remission increased as the time lapse between ratings became longer. It should be noted that the acting-out conduct problem dimension was consistently more stable than the personality problem dimension (Apathy-Withdrawal).

When preschool was the point of prediction, Apathy-Withdrawal was strongly associated with poor cognitive functioning and Anger-Defiance was less strongly related. When first grade was the point of prediction, Apathy-Withdrawal was related to educational failure on every criterion variable. With increasing age, social-emotional functioning and academic attainment both worsened.

Some stability of Factor I and Factor II dimensions were demonstrated across situations (school and residence in an institution for delinquent children), but at best the correlations accounted for 36 percent of the variance (.40 for Factor I and .60 for Factor II). Emotional impairment in preschool was considered to be predictive of later emotional impairment even after the demographic variables of social class, sex, and family intactness had been statistically controlled.

These findings were interpreted as demonstrating sufficient stability and predictiveness to enable identification of children at risk for subsequent emotional disturbance. However, it should be pointed out that the social-emotional variables accounted for only 16 to 27 percent of the variance of emotional impairment from preschool to the fourth grade and 23 to 33 percent of the variance from early to later elementary school.

Gersten et al. (1976, 1979) used data from a structured questionnaire obtained at two points approximately five years apart to investigate stability and change in types of behavior disturbance of children and adolescents. They derived six factors representing types of disturbances: mentation problems, fighting, conflict with parents, regressive anxiety, isolation, and delinquency. The three dimensions reflecting aggressive or antisocial behaviors (fighting, conflict with parents, and delinquency) either increased in the pathological direction or remained relatively constant within a five-year period, while the neurotic behaviors (mentation problems, regressive anxiety, and isolation) declined in disturbance with advancing age. For both types of problems, stability was high; that is, a child's placement relative to the group remained consistent.

Gersten et al. (1976, 1979) attempted to determine the age at which these dimensions of behavior problems had stabilized and consolidated (thereby having greater prognostic significance) and whether referrals at these points in time, as opposed to earlier or later, resulted in greater efficacy in decreasing the future risk. Their results demonstrated that the antisocial behavior of delinquency appeared to become an established pattern around ten years of age; the neurotic behavior of regressive anxiety at middle adolescence; and mentation problems, fighting, and conflict with parents before and into latency (six to nine years of age). No prediction was possible for isolation because there was no sharp increase in stability with age. However, for none of the types of disturbance did the referral rates differ among the age cohorts. Furthermore, across all types of disturbances, the referred children had rates of future pathology equal to or greater than nonreferred children. The results regarding differential effectiveness based on age of referral for types of problem received partial support. The results were confirmatory for anxiety- or neurotic-type problems and for mentation problems and for the prediction of no differential effectiveness for isolative-withdrawn types. The results for conflicts with parents were consistent with expectations but not for fighting and delinquency. With delinquency, evidence was provided for the consolidation but not for the differential effectiveness of referral at this point. Consistent with other studies (Robins 1966), antisocial behavior in adolescence was predictive of adult antisocial behavior, and those referred for treatment at these adolescent ages had a risk of future impairment that was nearly three times greater than those not referred.

In their review, Achenbach and Edelbrock (1978) indicate that children manifesting the Overcontrolled-internalizing and the Undercontrolled-externalizing syndromes were very different children living in very different families. In terms of the children, within-sex comparisons have generally shown that internalizers adapt better than externalizers as reflected in school performance, scores on standardized tests, and teacher and peer ratings, and they remain longer in, and improve more from, psychotherapy (Achenbach and Lewis 1971). Externalizers have been shown to be more impulsive and have less self-control on measures of delay of gratification, reflection-impulsivity, and foresight (Weintraub 1973). In terms of parents, those of internalizers have been found to be more strict with their children and more concerned about the problems of the child. They also have fewer marital separations and social problems, and less overall pathology than parents of externalizers (Achenbach and Edelbrock 1978). Achenbach and Edelbrock concluded that "undercontrolled children and their families are in more open conflict with other people, are less socially competent, and are less appropriate candidates for traditional mental health services" (pp. 1293–94).

## Childhood Behavior Problems and Subsequent Adjustment

Robins (1978) studied a diverse sample of males and found that every type of childhood antisocial behavior predicted a high level of adult antisocial behavior, and that each type of adult antisocial behavior was predicted by the number of childhood behaviors. Robins contends that these findings argue for the unitary nature of antisocial behavior in childhood and adulthood. The findings also confirmed: (1) that adult antisocial behavior virtually requires childhood antisocial behavior; (2) that most antisocial children do not become antisocial adults in that even highly antisocial children become highly antisocial adults in only 50 percent or fewer cases (thus, childhood antisocial behavior is a necessary but not sufficient condition for adult antisocial personality); (3) that the variety of antisocial behavior in childhood is a better predictor of antisocial behavior than is any particular behavior; and (4) that childhood behavior is a better predictor than family background or social class of rearing. Robins points out that these findings place an emphasis upon developing methods to identify the 50 percent of highly antisocial children who are at risk for being antisocial adults and to determine what accounts for the good outcome in the 50 percent who do not turn out to be antisocial adults. Also, the question arises as to how to intervene to prevent those who are at risk from being antisocial adults.

In another review, Robins (1979) examined follow-up studies of children's behavior disorders broadly defined as: reported symptoms, difficulties at school or with the law, or referral to a psychiatrist before age eighteen. Robins reports that autism, schizophrenia, and conduct problems are the categories of childhood psychopathology with which serious adult difficulties are associated. Contrary to common conceptions, the anxiety-withdrawal disorders of childhood have a rather good prognosis.

In their review of the predictability of adult mental health from childhood behavior, Kohlberg, LaCross, and Rick (1972) reach a similar conclusion. With the exception of schizophrenia and sociopathy, emotional disturbance in childhood is not seen as a useful predictor of adult mental health.

In summary, our review indicates the substantial challenge that confronts empirical approaches to the delineation and classification of children's behavior problems. While it is possible to differentiate referred children from normal children along a number of behavioral dimensions, the prevalence of behavior problems in the normal population is high and varies with age and sex. There is some stability of these dimensions but this decreases with increasing time between measurements, and with the exception of psychosis and antisocial behavior, there is insufficient consistency to predict subsequent adjustment. Even with antisocial behavior only 50 percent of those with highly antisocial behavior in childhood turn out to be highly antisocial adults.

In general, it has been determined that the externality syndrome is associated with more undesirable outcomes than the internality syndrome. The utility of these findings will be enhanced as methods are developed, such as cluster analysis, to translate scores on broad- and narrow-band dimensions into individual behavior profiles. The association of these behavior profiles with etiological and outcome variables can then be determined. Furthermore, increased efforts will need to be directed

toward formation of more homogeneous subgroups on the basis
of patterns of behavior disturbance.

## Social Relationships of Children with Behavior Problems

Up to this point the discussion has focused primarily upon parent
and teacher ratings of the behavior of children as the empirical
basis for identifying patterns of behavior problems and their
relative frequencies. An alternate line of empirical investigation
has been the use of peer nominations to identify children with
specific types of behavior patterns—for example, aggressive,
withdrawn, rejected—and those at risk for subsequent psychopathology. Peer nominations have also been used to gather information about the social relationships of children with learning
and/or behavioral problems. Frequently, sociometric studies are
combined with observational or laboratory study of the social
interactions of target groups with peers and adults.

Ledingham has conducted a series of studies designed to
identify children who are at high risk for schizophrenia and has
used peer ratings to delineate patterns of behavioral problems.
Ledingham (1981) obtained peer ratings on a French translation
of the Pupil Evaluation Inventory (Pekarik et al. 1976) from a
total of 4,110 children in grades one, four, and seven in French-
language schools in Montreal. The Pupil Evaluation Inventory
contains thirty-five items that load on three factors: aggression,
withdrawal, and likeability. Z scores on the aggression and withdrawal factors were used to select target subjects. Children with
Z scores > ninety-fifth percentile on aggression and < seventy-
fifth percentile on withdrawal were designated as aggressive.
Children with Z scores > ninety-fifth percentile on withdrawal
and < seventy-fifth percentile on aggression were designated as
withdrawn. Those with Z scores > seventy-fifth percentile on
both aggression and withdrawal were designated aggressive-
withdrawn. Control children had Z scores < seventy-fifth percentile on both aggression and withdrawal. In addition to peer
ratings, following the selection of target subjects 105 teachers

rated the current behavior of 64 aggressive, 67 withdrawn, 77 aggressive-withdrawn, and 146 controls using a French translation of the Devereaux Elementary School Behavior Rating Scale (DESD) (Spivack and Swift 1967). Data are also reported for mother ratings of a French translation of the Devereaux Child Behavior Rating Scale (Spivack and Spotts 1966) for 179 target and control children.

The findings indicated that peer likeability ratings in grade one were higher than those in grades four and seven across all groups. The aggressive-withdrawn group had significantly lower likeability scores than did the aggressive and control groups and had signficantly lower likeability scores than the withdrawn group at grades one and seven.

In terms of teacher ratings there were significant group effects on ten out of the eleven scales of the Devereaux. The aggressive and aggressive-withdrawn groups were rated significantly higher than the withdrawn and control groups on: classroom disturbance, impatience, disrespect-defiance, external blame, irrelevant responses, and tendency to give up on tasks. Control subjects were also rated as significantly more disturbing to the class than withdrawn subjects. The three target groups were rated lower on comprehension than were the controls. Withdrawn subjects were rated significantly lower on the creative initiative scale than were the aggressive, aggressive-withdrawn, and control groups. The aggressive-withdrawn group was described as more externally reliant, more inattentive-withdrawn, less able to change tasks easily, and slower to complete work than the other groups. Thus, by demonstrating differences among groups across the behavior dimensions, the teacher ratings provided support for the distinctiveness of the groups initially determined by peer nominations. That is, aggressive, aggressive-withdrawn, and withdrawn groups were lower on comprehension than were the controls; aggressive and aggressive-withdrawn were higher on aggression than the withdrawn and control groups; and the withdrawn and aggressive-withdrawn groups were higher on withdrawal than aggressive and control groups.

Mothers ratings also provided support for the peer-determined groups. Mothers rated the aggressive and aggressive-withdrawn groups higher than the withdrawn and control groups on social aggression and unethical behavior. The withdrawn and aggressive-withdrawn groups were also rated higher on emotional detachment, proneness to emotional upset, and inability to delay than were the aggressive and control groups. Furthermore, the withdrawn group was rated significantly higher on social isolation than were the aggressive, aggressive-withdrawn, and control groups; and the aggressive group was rated higher on pathological use of senses and needing less adult contact than the withdrawn, aggressive-withdrawn, or control groups. The aggressive-withdrawn subjects were described as taking poorer care of themselves than the withdrawn subjects, and as more distractible, as making more pathological use of their senses, and as needing more adult contact than all other groups.

Both teacher and parent ratings indicated that the aggressive-withdrawn group was deviant in comparison not only to the control group but also to the aggressive and withdrawn groups as well. Ledingham (1981) concluded that children who are both aggressive and withdrawn are less mature and less socially skilled and are thus potenially at risk for subsequent poor adjustment.

To assess the hypothesized risk potential, a follow-up study was done three years subsequently of 122 children from the aggressive group, 150 from the withdrawn group, 182 from the aggressive-withdrawn group, and 299 control-group children (Ledingham and Schwartzman 1984). School progress was adopted as an intermediate outcome measure for children believed to be at risk behaviorally for later psychopathology. The children's educational placement was classified as "regular class at expected grade level" or as "school difficulty," comprising those in regular class but at least one grade below expected grade level and children in special education class both at and below expected grade level. The frequency of school difficulty was compared across the behavioral subgroup classification. The findings indicated that boys did more poorly at follow-up than girls, with 65 percent of the boys in regular class at expected grade level versus 74 percent of the girls. However, there was a significant relationship across sex and grade between behavioral subgroup classification and school placement at follow-up. There were fewer aggressive-group children (5 percent) and aggressive-withdrawn group children (52 percent) in regular class at expected grade level than withdrawn group children (75 percent) and control group children (83 percent). Special class placement below grade level occurred for 12 percent of the aggressive-withdrawn group, 7 percent of the aggressive group, 2 percent of the withdrawn group, and for no control group children. The major finding was that aggressive children experienced more difficulties in school than withdrawn or control children and the aggressive-withdrawn children had the poorest academic adaptation.

The studies by Ledingham demonstrated that peer ratings can delineate children into subgroups on the basis of aggressive and withdrawn behavioral dimensions. It was also demonstrated that aggressive, withdrawn, and aggressive-withdrawn subgroups of children can be differentiated from each other and from controls on the basis of parent and teacher ratings and school performance. Again, evidence is provided for poor subsequent function for children characterized as aggressive, and some evidence was provided for the particular deviance and lower likeability of children who are both aggressive and withdrawn.

The importance and utility of using both positive and negative sociometric choice questions to obtain a more differentiated picture of a child's social status among his or her peer group has been demonstrated by Coie, Dodge, and Cappotelli (1982). A total of 311 third, fifth, and eighth grade students were administered a sociometric nomination interview and were asked to nominate three peers that they "like most" and "like least" and three peers who best fit each of twenty-four behavioral descriptions. To assess the correlates of "like most" and "like least," each of the twenty-four behavioral descriptions were correlated with these two scores. The major correlates of the "like most" score included: supports peers, attractive physically, cooperates with peers, and leads peers. The major correlates of the "like least" score included: disrupts the group, aggresses indirectly, starts fights, gets into trouble with teacher, and acts snobbish. Two additional sociometric variables were derived from the "like most" and "like least" scores. Social preference was calculated by subtracting the "like least" score from the "like most" score. Social impact was calculated by adding the two scores together. These dimensions of social status were subsequently used to form five different status types: popular, rejected, neglected (i.e., receiving few "like least" and no "like most" nominations), controversial (i.e., receiving high liking and high disliking scores), and average. Peer-perceived differences in behavior patterns among the five social status groups were also identified.

To obtain these behavioral descriptions from peers, the twenty-four-item instrument utilized previously was reduced, through hierarchical cluster analysis, to six items: cooperates, disrupts, shy, fights, seeks help, and leader. The data from the initial 311 subjects were combined with the data from 537 additional children. Of the total of 848 children, 486 were selected as fitting one of the social status types: 104 in the popular group, 111 in the rejected group, 112 in the neglected group, 62 in the controversial group, and 77 in the average group.

The popular group received high scores on "cooperativeness" and "leader" and low scores on "disrupts," "fights," and "seeks help." The rejected group received low scores on "cooperates" and "leader" but high scores on "disrupts," "fights," and "seeks help." The controversial children were perceived as disruptive, as starting fights, and as seeking help, but they were also perceived as leaders. The controversial children received scores similar to the average group in cooperation and below the mean on shyness. While the controversial group is a high visibility group, the neglected group is the polar opposite. These children are not aggressive, not leaders, low on cooperation, and somewhat shy. The authors point out that the controversial group is similar to the children described by Roff et al. (1972) who received large numbers of both positive and negative sociometric nominations and who appeared to be at risk for juvenile delinquency.

In two studies sociometric nominations were used to select groups of popular, average, rejected, and neglected third and fifth grade children (Dodge, Coie, and Brakke 1982). The peer interactions of these children were observed in their classrooms and on the playground. A six-category behavioral event coding system was utilized. Two categories described solitary activity (solitary task-appropriate and solitary task-inappropriate). Two described aggressive acts, with a distinction as to whether the child initiated or was the object of aggression. Two categories described prosocial approaches, with a distinction regarding initiation by subject or by peer, and if by a subject whether it was accepted or rejected by the peer. Teachers also rated the academic performance and social adjustment of each subject.

The findings indicated that rejected children initiated almost twice as many peer-directed aggressive acts as popular or average children. In contrast to the popular children, the rejected children demonstrated fewer task-appropriate behaviors and more aggressive behaviors and task-inappropriate behaviors. Rejected children prosocially approached peers as frequently as did popular children, but the peer responses were more likely to be negative toward rejected children. The neglected children demonstrated relatively few task-inappropriate and aggressive behaviors and they socially approached peers infrequently, but this behavior met with frequent rejection. The findings were discussed in terms of the need for different types of social-skill training by children with different types of social status.

In a series of studies summarized by Dodge (1985) aggressive boys, identified by classroom peers and by teachers, have been found consistently to differ from nonaggressive boys in social information processing. Aggressive boys demonstrate response-decision bias (generate a higher proportion of aggressive, incompetent solutions in response to hypothetical problems), hostile attributional bias (attribute hostile intent to the peer in ambiguous provocation circumstances), and cue-utilization deficiency (use irrelevant or fewer cues in making attributions).

Milich and Dodge (1984) studied these three social information processing deficits in a child psychiatric population subgrouped according to the fourfold model of hyperactivity identified by Loney and her colleagues (Loney, Langhorne, and Paternite 1978) which is discussed in a subsequent section. It was hypothesized that the information-processing deficits would be most pronounced for the combined hyperactive/aggressive subgroup. The clinic sample consisted of seventy-five boys divided into hyperactive/aggressive ($N = 24$), hyperactive ($N = 14$), aggressive ($N = 14$), and psychiatric control ($N = 23$) groups. A normal control group ($N = 60$) was composed of randomly selected boy classmates. The subjects participated in several tasks to solicit information-processing patterns. The findings indicated that the hyperactive-aggressive group was deficient in all three areas assessed relative to the normal control group. While not differing in their hostile attributional bias from the other psychiatric groups, the hyperactive-aggressive group was 60 percent more likely than the normal control groups and other psychiatric groups to decide that they would retaliate aggressively against the peer instigator of the provocation and were also deficient in cue utilization relative to the other psychiatric groups. By demonstrating that the hyperactive-aggressive group displays a unique and deviant pattern of processing social information, the findings of this study provide additional evidence that the hyperactive-aggressive group is a behaviorally deviant group.

Milich and Landau (1984) conducted a study to compare the social status and social behavior of aggressive and aggressive-withdrawn boys as proposed by Ledingham (1981). The subjects consisted of forty-nine boys attending five kindergarten classrooms with an age range of 68 to 84 months and a mean of 74.6 months. Teacher rankings of popularity were obtained along with teacher ratings on the Connors Teacher Rating Scale. Social behavior was assessed by observation of free play. Peer nominations yielded ten aggressive, nine withdrawn, ten aggressive-withdrawn, and twenty control children.

The findings indicated that peers rated the aggressive children as both popular and rejected (i.e., controversial) but rated the aggressive-withdrawn children as rejected. The teachers rated the aggressive and aggressive-withdrawn groups high on aggression and rated the aggressive-withdrawn group significantly higher than the other three groups on hyperactivity. The teacher rankings of popularity yielded results similar to those from the peer nomination of rejection—that is, the aggressive and the aggressive-withdrawn children had social status problems. In terms of observed social behavior, the withdrawn group was significantly higher on solitary play and the aggressive and aggressive-withdrawn groups were higher on observed negative interpersonal behavior. The aggressive group was also significantly high on observed positive interpersonal behavior. The authors note the similarity of their aggressive-withdrawn group to the hyperactive-aggressive group described by Loney and her colleagues and of the aggressive group to the controversial group described by Coie et al. (1982). That is, while the aggressive-withdrawn group is seen as rejected it is also rated as more than twice as hyperactive as any other group; the aggressive group is high in negative interpersonal behavior, positive interpersonal behavior, peer rejection, and aggression. We will consider the hyperactive dimension more fully in the subsequent section.

Summary

The two major lines of empirical investigation discussed in this monograph can be seen to converge. The factor analysis of behavior-problem ratings of parents and teachers demonstrate the existence of internalizing and externalizing behavior-problem patterns. Subsequent outcome difficulties are associated with the externalizing pattern. Factor-analytic studies of hyperactive children have delineated separate aggressive and hyperactive dimensions and revealed groups that are exclusively hyperactive, exclusively aggressive, and exclusively hyperactive and aggressive. Those that are hyperactive and aggressive appear to be social rejected by peers and to have the poorest outcome.

Social status types generated by peer nominations have consistently shown that peer nominated aggression is associated with adverse adult outcome, and that some youngsters are neglected, popular, rejected, and controversial (i.e., both rejected and popular). This leads to the recognition that the status of aggressive children on other dimensions such as popularity, social rejection, and withdrawal is necessary for appropriate risk assessment and development of effective intervention programs.

# CHAPTER 5

# Behavior Problems and Learning Disabilities

While the study of behavior problems has been hampered by the absence of well-delineated and measurable patterns of behavior disturbance, the study of behavior problems in children with learning problems has been hampered further by assumptions that: (1) a strong association exists between learning disorders and emotional disorders; (2) emotional or behavioral problems are the basis for the learning problems; and (3) a common pattern of personality or behavior problems is associated with learning problems.

For many years there was a tacit assumption that learning disorders and emotional problems were related. This assumption influenced diagnostic and intervention procedures. Clements and Peters (1962, 185) reported that for ". . . many years, it has been the custom among child guidance workers to attribute the behavior and learning deviations seen in children almost exclusively to the rearing patterns and interpersonal relations experienced by such youngsters. In many clinics, it has become habitual to assume psychogenicity when no easily recognizable organic deviation can be found."

Perhaps the reliance upon psychogenic theories occurred because of their capacity to explain phenomena and assuage one's lack of knowledge and understanding. The traditional psychoanalytic view interprets learning problems as resulting from failure to identify with parents and teacher (Connolly 1971, Jampolsky 1965). Klein (1949) has stressed the importance of the need for the infant's gratification in the first year of life as a necessary preparation for learning, while Sylvester and Kunst (1943) have emphasized the significance of the thwarting of the child's early exploratory activities on later reading problems. Those children who have not resolved their Oedipal conflict may be fearful of hostile and aggressive impulses and, therefore, be afraid to succeed or to be competitive and, thereby, demonstrate learning problems (Jampolsky 1965). The role of anxiety, stemming from intrapersonal and interpersonal conflict, in inhibiting children from learning has also been acknowledged (Jampolsky 1965). With marked impairment, the severely disturbed or schizophrenic child may be so involved in his own fantasy that he is unable to learn (Jampolsky 1965, Pearson 1955).

Although there has been a history of reliance upon psychogenic theories, evidence has now accumulated that illustrates the gross inadequacy of conceptualizing learning disorders as simply a manifestation of an underlying emotional disturbance (Connolly 1971). Because of the evidence of the influence of neurological factors as well as psychological factors in learning problems, "the inaccuracies and limitations of the traditional psychiatric framework have become apparent" (Connolly 1971, 154).

What has resulted is a more considered view. Some children with learning problems do exhibit neurotic fears and traits previously described in the psychodynamic literature. But it is no longer assumed that all or that most of the youngsters with learning problems fit into this conceptual framework. Some children fail to learn and exhibit behavior problems because of a primary emotional problem stemming from organic or environmental factors. For other children, the emotional problems are secondary and "the maladaptive behavior is best understood as a result of interplay of inadequately developed primary skill system and environmental stresses that interfere with psychosexual development, and adversely influence self-concept" (Rubin 1971, 182). The probability that a learning disabled child will develop emotional or behavioral problems is related to many variables such as severity and chronicity of the problem, age, sex, subcultural group, socioeconomic level, and intelligence (Connolly 1971). Many learning disabled children do cope well. However, all encounter serious obstacles to adjustment, and emotional demands and stress exceed those encountered by most other children.

Learning disabled children have the same basic needs and drives as other children, such as needs for acceptance, adequacy, competency, and mastery; but their handicap sometimes obstructs the satisfaction of these needs and drives. When this occurs, adjustment is threatened and emotional and behavior problems may develop. In 1971 Connolly (161) stated: "The literature is in almost unanimous agreement in stating that there is no single reaction pattern or syndrome of behavior common to the learning disabled population." However, more recently it has been contended that there is a link between learning disabilities and juvenile delinquency (Berman 1981).

A child with cognitive-perceptual-motor difficulties can be viewed as vulnerable (Rubin 1971). This vulnerability can lead to learning and behavior problems that influence the reaction of environmental figures. Frequently, these significant environmental figures (parents and teachers) can respond with blame and criticism that increases stress and feelings of frustration and tension. Poor self-concept results from failures and from the feedback that the child receives from others. This poor self-concept and feelings of inadequacy are likely to prolong dependency and immaturity and the utilization of immature defense mechanisms, such as projection of blame and avoidance. This avoidance of tasks impairs motivation and causes a further deficit in skills because certain skills must be practiced to be learned. Thus, there is a lack of improvement, which perpetuates this vicious circle.

Recently, there has been a reliance upon categorical models based upon an either/or theory of etiology, that is, conceptualizing school maladjustment either as a learning problem or as an emotional problem. This has resulted in some benefits such as classes designed for learning disabled and for emotionally disturbed children. However, the underlying continuum has been obscured. As Rubin stated, "the absence of a theoretical construct that permits integration of personality deviations and learning disability means that many children with disturbed behavioral functioning are misunderstood and mishandled" (Rubin 1971, 181).

What has been needed is a model that integrates an understanding of personality variables with other functional impairments. The model of secondary emotional problems as outlined above with its focus upon environmental factors interacting with vulnerabilities is one model that has had some heuristic value.

## Behavior Problems in Children with Learning Problems

A number of studies have been done with special-education populations that suggest that the factor structure of behavior problems in these special groups are very similar to those found in the general population and with other clinical subgroups. In addition, the majority of evidence indicates higher levels of behavior problems in these special populations as compared to controls but less than the levels demonstrated by youngsters with primary behavioral problems.

Quay and Gredler (1981) examined the factor structure of the BPC ratings of 252 institutionalized retarded persons (mean age = 21.8 years; mean IQ = 37.8). The broad-band dimensions of Conduct Disorder (CD) and Anxiety-Withdrawal (PP—Personality Problem) were represented, as well as a third factor reflecting psychotic behavior. However, scores on all of the BPC scales were well below those reported for various behaviorally disordered samples. These results were interpreted as indicating that the degree of psychopathology evidenced by this population was comparable to that for age-matched normals.

Grieger and Richards (1976) investigated the Behavior Problem Checklist (BPC) factor structure of 100 children from classes for the emotionally disturbed or learning disabled and 527 children from the regular first through seventh grade classrooms. The results yielded three factors for both the regular and special education subgroups that closely corresponded to the factors of Conduct Disorder, Personality Problems, and Inadequacy-Immaturity (II) that have been identified in many studies of children's behavior problems. Although the factor structure for the children from the special education classes was similar to that obtained from the children in the regular classes, the special education children scored higher on all three factors than their sex-and age-matched counterparts in the normal classroom. The authors point out that the percentage of behavioral symptoms in the regular-classroom children were remarkably similar to those reported by Werry and Quay (1971) for the general population.

In a study of 192 white and 17 Mexican-American children in special education classes and 1,999 white and 192 Mexican-American children in regular classrooms, Lindholm and Touliatos (1976) found that the children in the special education classes scored higher on all of the BPC factors than did the children in the regular classes. These results were significant for the white children but were not significant for the Mexican-American children.

In their review of studies using the BPC with educationally handicapped or clinically deviant children and nondeviant controls, Cullinan, Epstein, and Denbinski (1979) concluded that deviant groups differ from normals on some or all of the BPC dimensions of maladjustment and that there is some evidence that deviant subgroups vary among themselves. This question of whether the various subgroups of educationally handicapped children demonstrate different patterns of behavioral disorder has been one that has prompted considerable research.

Cullinan et al. (1979) examined the teacher BPC ratings of 104 learning disabled, behavior disordered, educably mentally retarded, and normal (not identified for special education class) male pupils aged six to eighteen years. Differences among the subgroups of children were obtained on a number of the BPC factors. On the Conduct Disorder factor, the behavior dis-

ordered children exceeded all other groups and the mentally
retarded (MR) group exceeded the normal group. On the Personality Problem factor, the behavior disordered and learning
disabled groups each exceeded the normal group. On the Inadequacy-Immaturity factor, the mentally retarded group exceeded
the normal group. Thus, the normal pupils could be distinguished from all categories of those requiring special education
on the basis of personality problems. Among the educationally
handicapped, the behaviorally disordered could be discrimi-
nated from the learning disabled and the mentally retarded on
the basis of conduct disorder problems. In this study, discrimination of the learning disabled and mentally retarded was not
possible. However, the mentally retarded group was significantly
higher on Conduct Disorder problems and on Inadequacy-
Immaturity than the normal children. The authors postulate that
personality problems differentiate between normal and handicapped groups, and conduct disorder problems differentiate behavior disordered from learning impaired (LD and MR) groups.

The study by Gajar (1979) also addressed the question of difference in behavior disorders as a function of subgroup of educational handicap. The BPC ratings of 122 emotionally disturbed,
135 learning disabled, and 121 educably mentally retarded children with respective group full-scale Wechsler Intelligence Scale
for Children-Revised (WISC-R) IQ means of 91.48, 91.67, and
70.14 were investigated. The emotionally disturbed group differed significantly from the mentally retarded and learning disabled groups on the Conduct Disorder and Personality Problem
factors and from the mentally retarded group on the Inadequacy-
Immaturity factor. All groups demonstrated a higher average
score on the Inadequacy-Immaturity factor than on the Conduct
Disorder and Personality Problem factors. These results differ
somewhat from those of McCarthy and Paraskevopoulos (1969).
In their study, thirty-six children with learning disabilities, one
hundred in special education classes for emotionally disturbed
children, and forty-one average children were involved. The
findings indicated that the emotionally disturbed children scored

higher than the learning disabled children, who scored higher than the average children, on the unsocialized Aggressive factor, Personality Problem factor, and the Inadequacy-Immaturity factor. This finding is consistent with others reported above in indicating more disturbance in emotionally disturbed than learning disabled children. However, both the emotionally disturbed and learning disabled group exhibited more Conduct Disorder problems than Inadequacy-Immaturity or Personality Problems.

In a study contrasting learning disabled children ($N = 16$) not with emotionally disturbed but with other clinical subgroups represented by epilepsy ($N = 16$) and hyperactivity ($N = 15$) as well as control children ($N = 50$), Campbell (1974) found that all clinical groups scored significantly higher on the Inadequacy-Immaturity factor than did the controls. The hyperactive children scored significantly higher on the Conduct Disorder factor than the control, epileptic, and learning disabled children. Furthermore, the epileptic children scored signficantly higher than the controls on Conduct Disorder problems as well.

Touliatos and Lindholm (1980) examined behavior disorders of learning disabled ($N = 94$) and normal ($N = 2,991$) children in grades kindergarten through eight. The learning disabled children had significantly more problems on Personality Problem, Conduct Disorder, and Inadequacy-Immaturity factors and on psychotic signs, but not on the Socialized Delinquency factor, than normals. It was interesting to note that the frequency of personality problem syndromes increased steadily for the learning disabled group across grades, while they increased for normal subjects from kindergarten to grades two to three and then declined. Including this type of developmental perspective is crucial to fostering our knowledge about the point at which intervention programs need to be instituted. For example, if we know that personality problems are frequent in normal children up to grade three but decrease thereafter, persistence of problems past that point would be "atypical" and perhaps unlikely to remit without intervention.

Finally, the efforts to document the existence of similar dimensions of behavioral problems in various educational, clinical, and normal populations has been extended to a consideration of youngsters with educational problems of such a nature that allowed the children to be mainstreamed (Larrivee and Bourque 1981). In this study, the factor structure of behavior problems was examined using teacher ratings on the Devereaux Elementary School Rating Scale (DESD) (Spivack and Swift 1967) of 146 mainstreamed students requiring special education programming in kindergarten to sixth grade. The findings for the total group extracted five factors: three representing the familiar Personality Problem, Conduct Problem, and Inadequacy-Immaturity factors reported in other studies, as well as two additional factors that reflected the inclusion of items relating specifically to the demands of the classroom environment. These two factors were achievement anxiety and adaptive classroom behavior. The congruence in factor structure between the mainstreamed and regular classroom students was high for the factors of Conduct Disorder, Personality Problem, adaptive classroom behavior, and achievement anxiety, and less high for Inadequacy-Immaturity.

In summary, a number of studies have utilized behavior checklists to assess the nature and extent of behavior problems in populations of children with educational problems, ranging from those requiring special educational programs to those that are mainstreamed. The findings indicate that the factor structure of behavior problems in these special groups is very similar to that found in the general population and in other clinical subgroups: Personality Problem, Conduct Problem, and Inadequacy-Immaturity factors. Most studies report that the special education subgroups have higher levels of all three behavior problem factors than normal control children. In addition, contrasts are frequently made with respect to the extent of behavior problems among subgroups of children requiring special education, such as children with mental retardation, learning problems, and emotional problems. The findings are not always consistent with respect to the relative frequencies of each of the three factors. However, the studies do reveal higher levels of behavioral disturbance among children with emotional problems than among those with primary learning problems (LD and MR). Those with primary learning problems demonstrate higher levels of behavioral disturbance than normal controls, but differences between the MR and LD subgroups are inconsistently reported.

## Learning Disability and Juvenile Delinquency: Evidence of a Link?

There has been a resurgence of interest in the possibility of a link between learning disabilities and juvenile delinquency (JD). In part, this stems from an appreciation of the fact that many children who were or are adjudicated have learning and school performance difficulties. In a comprehensive review, Berman (1981) remarked: "Despite the early and continued findings of an association linking learning disorders to delinquency, there still is much resistance to the idea that the two are significantly related . . ." (p. 245). Berman postulated several reasons for the controversy surrounding such a link, among which he included definitional and methodological problems and psychodynamic heritage.

The definitional problems with juvenile delinquency are similar to those previously discussed concerning learning disabilities and behavior problems. That is, there is a lack of an accepted operational definition. Most frequently the determination of delinquency rests on whether a youngster has been adjudicated by a court; however, delinquency is sometimes determined by a self-report of behavior that may or may not have come to the attention of the courts. Some studies employ only institutionalized delinquents while others use unincarcerated delinquents.

Methodologically, the most frequently found problems include a lack of appropriate control groups and a reliance upon retrospective designs. In reviewing the evidence for the link between learning disabilities and juvenile delinquency, Spreen (1981) notes that retrospective designs almost inevitably result in finding a strong relationship between a precursor and subsequent problem. Prospective designs, on the other hand, suggest that a majority of children demonstrating the precursor do *not* develop the subsequent problem hypothesized to be associated with the precursor.

Mention has already been made of the impact of the psychodynamic heritage noted by Berman (1981). That is, both learning problems and delinquency are viewed as being of psychogenic origin. There is no doubt that in some situations learning problems and delinquency can be of psychogenic origin. However, in reviewing his own work and that of others, Berman contends that "there is considerable data (Berman 1972, 1974; Berman and Siegel 1976b) indicating that no psychogenic problems could be discerned in most LD children prior to the onset of school failure, and that later behavioral problems are a result of, not the cause of, failure related to their learning disabilities (see also Richardson, Brutten, and Nagel 1973; Levy 1973; Smith 1976)" (Berman 1981, 246).

Even large-scale government-initiated reviews and studies such as that by Murray (1976) (conducted through the American Institute for Research and the National Research and Demonstration Project), reviewed by Berman (1981) and Lane (1980), continue the controversy about the evidence for the link but do have heuristic value in addressing both content and methodological issues.

It is beyond the scope of this monograph to review adequately all the research evidence regarding the link between learning disability and juvenile delinquency. Several studies are presented that will illustrate the divergence of samples, methods, and findings that currently characterize the research literature concerning the LD-JD link.

A study done by Robbins et al. (1983) focused upon the neuropsychological status of unincarcerated male delinquents. There were two primary questions: (1) Are unincarcerated male delinquents neuropsychologically impaired?; (2) Did neuropsychologically impaired delinquents differ from unimpaired delinquents in criminal history, social background, and physical and psychiatric status? The sample consisted of fifty boys, fourteen to eighteen years of age who were adjudicated, twenty-five of whom had been referred by a judge to a psychiatric clinic because evaluation and/or treatment was considered useful, and twenty-five nonclinic referred. The authors report that both the clinic and nonclinic subgroups of those adjudicated but unincarcerated delinquents were found to be significantly impaired on cognitive, perceptual, and perceptual-motor functions, with a number of indicators of minor neurological instabilities. While there was no difference between clinic and nonclinic groups in IQ, academic achievement, or in percentage occurrence of LD (ten out of twenty-five in the clinic group versus twelve out of twenty-five in the nonclinic group), there was a significant difference in auditory perception difficulties, visual problems, and Bender-Gestalt performance in favor of the nonclinic sample. In addition, there were more repeat offenders in the clinic sample. This study is representative of other studies that do not employ a control group but report positive test findings of neuropsychological impairment or dysfunction with samples of delinquents (unincarcerated males in this instance).

A study by Broder et al. (1981) did employ a control group and well-defined criteria for determination of the occurrence of LD in adjudicated delinquent boys. The sample consisted of 1,617 boys twelve to fifteen years of age. Of these, 620 were adjudicated delinquents and 968 had no records of adjudication. Determination of LD was primarily based on WISC-R and achievement test scores. If the child had test scores at or above the expected grade level for age on achievement test or a full scale intelligence quotient (FSIQ) greater than two standard deviations below the mean then the child was classified as not LD. A child was classified as LD if any three of the following criteria were met: (1) two years or greater discrepancy among WISC-R factors: analytic functioning, verbal comprehension, or attention; (2) two years or greater discrepancy among WISC-R factor scores and achievement scores or between achievement scores; (3) Bender-Gestalt score of three or more; (4) two or more ratings of pronounced difficulties on behavioral observations made by testers. The findings indicated that 36.5 percent of the adjudicated delinquents were LD compared to 18.9 percent of the control group. Of all the children classified as LD, 39.4 percent were delinquent.

Berman and Siegal (1976a, 1976b) administered the Halstead-Reitan Neuropsychology Battery to forty-five residents between the ages of fifteen and eighteen of the Rhode Island Training School, a detention facility for delinquents, and to forty-five students from two Providence high schools matched on the basis of age, race, sex, reading level, and socioeconomic status. None of the control students were "uncaught delinquents" and none were considered behavior problems by anyone who knew them. All training school students were serving their first sentence. The results indicated that, of the delinquent group, 70.1 percent scored in the impaired range on at least one of the Halstead-Reitan subtests, and 56 percent on at least two of the subtests. In the control group, 23 percent scored in the impaired range on one subtest and 18 percent on two or more subtests. In commenting on these findings Berman (1981, 262) remarked:

> While not meaning to imply that all LD children will necessarily become delinquent, the findings strongly support an argument that LD children are twice as likely to become delinquents as non-LD children, and that the experience of being LD leads to a cycle that may predispose the LD child to a greater degree of experience precipitating a delinquent lifestyle.

Spreen (1981) reported findings from a prospective follow-up study of 154 or 203 children who, between the ages of eight and twelve, had been referred for neuropsychological testing because of learning problems. The children with learning problems were followed up between four and twelve years later. At the time of original referral they were assessed as belonging to one of three diagnostic groups based on neurological examination: (1) fifty-two with definite neurological indications of brain damage;

(2) sixty-eight with neurological indications of suggested brain dysfunction; and (3) thirty-four learning disabled children without any neurological indications of brain dysfunction. A control group of fifty-two children without learning problems was randomly selected from secondary schools and matched with the three learning problem subgroups on age, sex, and socioeconomic level. At follow-up, separate interviews were conducted with subjects and one or both of the parents. The subjects and their parents were asked, "Have you ever come to the attention of the police?" The charges and penalties were also ascertained. The results indicated that 55 percent of the total sample had come to the attention of the police, but there were no significant differences between the learning impaired groups and the control group. The total number of first offenders did not differ significantly between groups, but there was a signficant difference in type of first offense. Vehicle-driving offenses were more frequent in the control group. Similarly, there were very few significant differences between groups in the frequencies of second, third, and fourth or subsequent offenses, nor in the type of these offenses. In terms of penalties, learning disabled children tended to receive slightly more and somewhat more severe penalties than the other groups.

While the studies reviewed are representative, they are not inclusive. What is essential for the purposes of this monograph is to recognize that a link has been postulated and to note the conflicting evidence. Even more germane to the focus of this monograph is to elucidate the relevant conceptual issues. One issue is that the postulation of a link focuses attention upon one type of behavior-problem pattern — externalizing-acting out-conduct disorder — being linked to learning disability. Our own research, to be discussed later, on delineating subgroup patterns of behavior problems should and can address this issue. Another conceptual issue germane to this monograph is the variety of models postulated to underlie the LD-JD link, three of which have been identified here. Berman (1981) points out that in one model there is an effort to relate brain damage to delinquency based on the relationship between brain damage and learning disability: "The rationale is that it is the LD and consequent educational problems that connect brain damage and delinquency" (Berman 1981, 249). Lane (1980) discusses the two models of the LD-JD link reflected in Murray's (1976) American Institute for Research Project. The susceptibility model views learning disabilities as accompanied by attributes of impulsivity, poor reception of social cues, and poor ability to learn from experience, which results in an increased susceptibility to juvenile delinquency. The school failure model views learning disabilities as causing school failure, which leads to a negative view of the child by adults, his or her peers, and by the child himself or herself, and then leads to association with a delinquent peer group.

Several comments are in order. While it is one thing to maintain that brain damaged individuals have learning problems, it is quite another to say that individuals with learning problems are brain damaged. The logic problem is one of reversibility of statements. Thus, if it is shown that most delinquents have learning problems, this does not affirm that most children with learning problems will be delinquent. Another point addresses the specificity of outcome postulated in the susceptibility and school failure models. Are not other types of behavior patterns, such as inhibition or withdrawal, just as likely an outcome as delinquency? What determines externalizing, internalizing, or behavior-problem-free outcomes in children with learning disabilities?

## Subtypes of Learning Disability

Just as it has been recognized that children with behavior problems are not a homogeneous group, it has also been recognized that children with learning disabilities are not a homogeneous group. The efforts at subgroup identification have focused upon common patterns of deficits or processing difficulties in children with learning disabilities (Leong 1982; Satz and Morris 1981) and on the overlap of learning disabilities with hyperactive behavior and with behavior problems. Recently, McKinney (1984) reviewed some of the research that began with a clinical inferential approach to subtypes and has now moved to multivariate hierarchical cluster-analytic techniques involving use of neuropsychological and psychoeducational test batteries. Cluster analysis involves correlation between subjects rather than between tasks, as in traditional factor analysis, and matches children according to their pattern of responses across an array of variables to form homogeneous subgroups with little overlap (Everitt 1980). Hierarchical cluster analysis is a technique that we have utilized in our efforts to delineate subgroups of children on the basis of patterns of behavior problems, which will be presented in a subsequent section of the monograph.

Of particular relevance to this monograph are the efforts to delineate subtypes of children with learning disabilities according to dimensions of behavior. These efforts have focused on: (1) differentiating subgroups of learning disabilities on the basis of presence or absence of hyperactivity and within hyperactivity based on aggressive behavior; and (2) on the inclusion of behavioral dimensions along with intellectual and academic dimensions in hierarchical cluster-analytic efforts at subtype formation.

## Hyperactivity

The terms *hyperactivity* and *learning disabilities* have been described as "two of the most troublesome terms in the field of child behavior disorders" (Lahey et al. 1978, 333). In contrast to the field of behavior problems, where factor analytic studies provide much support for the conduct problem and personality problem dimensions, little support has been provided for learning disabilities or hyperactivity as factors or dimensions of behavior. Lahey et al. (1978) postulated that this was because of the use of restricted item pools that contained few items relevant to these dimensions. They constructed a 110-item scale that included items designed to measure learning disabilities and hyperactivity. Nineteen teachers rated 404 children from special education and regular classes in grades two through eight. The results indicated four factors that were labeled conduct problems, personality problems, learning disabilities, and hyperactivity. These four factors were largely independent and accounted for 34.5 percent of the variance. While providing support for the inclusion of hyperactivity and learning disability as dimensions of behavior problems, the authors recognized that the diagnostic category of learning disabilities may constitute two or more behavioral subtypes. For example, while it can be argued that hyperactivity and learning disability are independent dimensions, most children who are hyperactive are likely to experience learning problems, and a high portion of children diagnosed as learning disabled are also likely to be diagnosed as hyperactive. However, not all those diagnosed as learning disabled are likely to be hyperactive. Similarly the diagnosis of hyperactivity typically involves not just overactivity, but specifically, overactivity that is inappropriate or leads to conflict with the child's environment. Lahey et al. (1978) point out that the diagnosis of hyperactivity may actually be applied to those who show deviations on both dimensions of hyperactivity and conduct problems. Differentiation of subgroups along these dimensions is essential if the effects of intervention are to be appropriately appreciated. For example, such differentiation enables the determination of whether the results of drug and behavioral treatment studies are due to effects on conduct problems or due to effects on hyperactivity.

Aggression

A major advance in subgroup delineation among children demonstrating the hyperkinetic/minimal brain dysfunction syndrome (MBD) has been made by Loney and her colleagues Langhorne, Paternite, and Beckholdt, and the University of Iowa.

In an early study Langhorne et al. (1976) found, as others had previously, little relationship among behavioral, cognitive, neurological, and medical history components in efforts to use factor analysis to identify syndrome subgroups in children with MBD. In their factor-analytic study of eleven often-cited core behavioral symptoms in ninety-four hyperkinetic boys, variables tended to cluster by source rather than symptom. While these results could be considered as indicating that MBD or hyperkinesis is not homogeneous, Langhorne et al. (1976) offered an alternative explanation that source factors result because the behavior of hyperkinetic children is different in different environments. This led to a search for factors among symptoms by analyzing data separately by source.

Loney et al. (1978) undertook a principal-axis factor analysis of the medical-chart ratings of primary and secondary symptoms. The subjects were 135 nonretarded, four to twelve-year-old hyperkinetic/MBD boys seen for outpatient diagnostic evaluations at the Child Psychiatry Service of the University of Iowa. Fifteen symptoms were rated by two judges. These consisted of six primary symptoms (hyperactivity, inattention, fidgetiness, judgment deficits or impulsivity, negative affect, and uncoordination); four secondary symptoms (compulsivity, aggressive interpersonal behavior, control deficits, and self-esteem deficits); and five unclassified marker symptoms (anxiety, depression, mood lability, speech disturbance, and sleep disturbance). Two variables, compulsivity and mood lability, were excessively skewed and were dropped, leaving thirteen variables for subsequent analysis. Two relatively independent symptom dimensions emerged: aggression, accounting for 44.6 percent of the factor variance, and hyperactivity, accounting for 23.4 percent of the factor variance. Correlations between factor scores on these dimensions and descriptors from parent and teacher rating scales provided evidence for concurrent validity. Higher scores on the aggression factor dimension were associated with (correlation significant $p < .05$) increased parent endorsement of descriptors such as: inconsiderate, cruel, quick-tempered, resentful, impertinent, won't mind, and resents authority. The aggression factor dimension was also associated with increased teacher endorsement of descriptors such as: destructive, defiant, teases other children or interferes with their activities, sullen or sulky, stubborn, quarrelsome, attendance problem, acts "smart," temper outbursts, impudent, and less likely as appearing too easily led. Higher scores on the hyperactivity factor dimension were associated with: increased parent endorsement of the descriptor impulsive and with increased teacher endorsement of the descriptors excessive demand for teacher's attention, restless/overactive, teases other children or interferes with their activities, tattles, disturbs other children, group does not seem to accept him, inattentive, less likely to be accepted by the group, or appears to be a leader. Based on these results, the authors postulated a fourfold model of hyperkinetic/MBD boys—those with: (1) low aggression and high hyperactivity (hyperactives); (2) high aggression and low hyperactivity (aggressives); (3) high aggression and high hyperactivity (aggressive hyperactives); and (4) low aggression and low hyperactivity (residuals).

Using the fourfold model, Langhorne and Loney (1979) investigated the direct and interactive effects of aggression and hyperactivity dimensions on a set of measures obtained at referral, during treatment with methylphenidate, and at a subsequent five-year follow-up in a group of eighty-four boys from the hyperactivity project at the University of Iowa. The boys in the sample were six to twelve years of age at the outpatient evaluation and twelve to eighteen years of age at follow-up. The results showed main effects for aggression and for hyperactivity on a number of dependent measures, but in no instance were there main effects for both factors on the same variable, nor were there any significant interactions. Significant main effects for the aggression factor indicated that more aggressive-hyperkinetic children come from lower SES homes and have parents who are rated as less loving, and the high-aggressive groups had fewer soft signs and lower self-esteem. Significant main effects for the hyperactive factor indicated that the high-hyperactive group made more errors on the Bender-Gestalt Test and were rated as demonstrating more initial drug response.

Delamater and colleagues have reported two studies of hyperactivity involving measures of autonomic activity. In one study Delamater, Lahey, and Drake (1981) investigated differences between hyperactive and nonhyperactive children on a number of tonic and phasic measures of autonomic activity. Hyperactivity was determined by teacher nominations and ratings on the Conner Teacher Rating Scale (CTRS). The hyperactive group (HA) consisted of eighteen males and three females with a mean age of 122 months; the nonhyperactive group (NHA) consisted of thirteen males and two females with a mean age of 119 months. The two groups did not differ on measures of skin conductance level, frequency of nonspecific skin conductance responses, or heart rate, nor on measures of skin conductance response amplitude to tones during the habituation task or on skin conductance latency. Thus, there were no significant differences between the groups on tonic and phasic measures of autonomic activity.

This study was followed by another one that used the same sample. In light of the evidence that aggression or conduct disorder may be a significant dimension for forming subgroups among hyperactive children, Delamater and Lahey (1983) designed a study to test the hypothesis that subgroups of hyperactive and learning disabled children defined by behavioral criteria will differ on physiological measures of arousal and responsiveness. Subjects consisted of thirty-six LD children of whom twenty-one were hyperactive and fifteen nonhyperactive. Subjects were subgrouped according to teacher ratings on the CTRS of tension anxiety and conduct problems. Subgroup comparisons were then made on measures of tonic and phasic autonomic arousal. Results indicated that subgroup formation among the overall sample of LD children on the basis of high or low conduct-problem dimension scores provided evidence of physiological heterogeneity. Children rated high on the conduct-problem dimension demonstrated smaller amplitude specific skin conductance responses than those low on conduct problems. Anxiety, as reflected in ratings on the tension-anxiety dimension, appeared to moderate the effect of conduct problems.

There was more difference in physiological measures between high and low subgroups on conduct problems with children who were rated low on tension-anxiety. When only the hyperactive sample was considered, those high on conduct problem evidenced significantly lower skin conductance levels than those low on conduct problems. However, since there were more blacks in the high conduct-problem subgroups the results are confounded with racial differences in electrodermal activity. Thus, these results are suggestive but inconclusive. However, across all physiological measures, the conduct-problem, low tension-anxiety subgroup demonstrated the lowest autonomic arousal (although not statistically significant in every case). The authors point out that these results are consistent with other research findings in showing that the presence of chronic aggression is associated with lower autonomic activity and later maladjustment in hyperactive children. In addition to providing some evidence that LD children are heterogeneous at a physiological level, the authors state that their findings suggest that physiological differences previously attributed to hyperactivity may actually be correlates of the conduct-problem dimension.

Behavior and Cognitive Dimensions

McKinney (1984) reasoned that behavior patterns would contribute to the definition of LD subtypes and therefore included a measure of classroom behavior—the Classroom Behavior Inventory (CBI) (Schaefer 1981)—in a hierarchical cluster-analytic study of fifty-nine school-defined first and second grade LD children. The CBI provides teacher ratings of academic competence, task orientation versus distractibility, extroversion versus introversion, and considerateness versus hostility. Also included were measures of intellectual ability (WISC-R) and educational achievement (Peabody Individual Achievement Test). Four subtypes of LD children were obtained. Subtype I represented 33 percent of the sample and was characterized by average verbal skills with deficits in sequential and spatial skills and deficiencies in independence and task-orientation. Subtype II represented 10 percent of the sample and characterized children with the highest scatter on the WISC-R, who were severely impaired in achievement, and were seen as less considerate, more hostile, less competent academically, and more poorly task-oriented than LD children in other subgroups. Subtype III included 47 percent of the sample and was distinguished by above average conceptual skills. These children were extroverted, but undifferentiated from normal comparison children in this regard, and were seen as less considerate and more hostile than other LD subgroups. Subtype IV consisted of 10 percent of the sample in whom there was no evidence of behavioral deficiency but who were more impaired in achievement than subtypes I or III.

While additional validation data is needed to determine the utility of McKinney's clusters of LD subtypes, including behavioral as well as academic and intellectual dimensions in the efforts to delineate subgroups would appear to offer the opportunity for specificity of intervention in terms of both behavioral as well as educational components.

## Social Relationships of Children with Learning Disabilities

The work of Tanis Bryan and her colleagues is representative of the use of observational studies and peer nominations to investigate the social relationships of learning disabled children. There are several reviews of Bryan's series of studies that reflect the systematic sequence of research questions prompting the studies (see Bryan, T. H., 1978, Bryan, J. H., 1981). The essential findings from these studies indicate that learning disabled children have difficulties in their social relationships with both peers and with teachers.

Observational studies (Bryan 1974a; Bryan and Wheeler 1972) have demonstrated that learning disabled children and peers spent the same amount of time interacting with peers and teachers but were twice as likely as comparison children to be

ignored by peers and teachers. While receiving the same number
of positive reinforcements from teachers, learning disabled children were also given twice as many negative reinforcements
from teachers as comparison subjects.

Bryan (1974b, 1978) has investigated the status or popularity
of learning disabled children with sociometric measures. Children completed a twenty-item questionnaire that asked them to
name children who are friends, who is handsome or pretty, who
you do not want to sit next to in class, etc. The scale yielded a
measure of social attraction and a measure of social rejection.
Learning disabled children received significantly more votes on
social rejection and significantly fewer votes on social attraction
than comparison children. White LD girls were the most rejected
of all. The children in this study were followed longitudinally,
with LD children again receiving more votes on rejection and
fewer votes on the attraction scale than comparison children,
even in classes in which the composition had changed more than
75 percent over the previous year.

The use of sociometric ratings by Bryan resulting in measures
of peer attraction and rejection enables subgroup formation by
considering a child's relative placement on each dimension.
Popular children are those below the group mean on rejection
and above the mean in attraction. Salient children score above
the group means on both attraction and rejection. Rejected
children score above the mean on rejection and below the mean
on attraction. Isolated children receive few scores from their
classmates on either the rejection and attraction scales. Bryan
(1977) suggested that the social interaction difficulties of children with learning disabilities may reflect a deficit in the comprehension of nonverbal communication. It was postulated that
nonverbal behavior requires the same basic learning processes—
such as attention and visual and auditory discrimination—that
are involved in learning to read. Thus, children who have difficulty learning to read may also have difficulty understanding
nonverbal behavior.

To evaluate this hypothesis Bryan (1977) employed the Profile of Nonverbal Sensitivity (PONS), an audio and video technique for assessing a child's understanding of nonverbal communication (Rosenthal et al. 1977, 1979). The test was given to eleven control children and twenty-three children who had been labeled by the school as having learning disabilities that warranted special education services from learning disability specialists. The children were in third, fourth, and fifth grade classrooms. The findings indicated that both groups obtained lower accuracy scores on the audio presentations than on the video presentations. The learning disabled children obtained a lower mean accuracy score than the control children ($p < .001$) and scored lower than the control children on both the audio and video presentations. However, there was an interaction effect between group and difficulty level of the presentation. The control and learning disabled children differed most on the easy audio items and the difficult video items.

Bryan (1977) acknowledges that the findings of the study do not permit analyses of the source of the group differences in understanding of nonverbal comprehension. The suggestion is made that less accurate comprehension of nonverbal communication by children with learning disabilities may be a specific aspect of their social relationships, which in turn affects both the reaction of others toward them and their social interaction behaviors.

Stone and La Greca (1984) conducted a study that was a partial replication and extension of Bryan's (1977) work that found LD children to be less accurate in comprehending nonverbal affective expression. Stone and La Greca (1984) attempted to determine whether learning disabled (LD) children differed from children not learning disabled (NLD) in their ability to comprehend nonverbal communication when potential attentional differences between the groups were controlled. The relationship between nonverbal comprehension and social competence was assessed through teacher's ratings of aggression and withdrawn behavior using the BPC and by judges' ratings of performance in a role-play of friendship-making skills. As in the

Bryan study (1977), nonverbal communication sensitivity was assessed using the PONS (Rosenthal et al. 1977, 1979), which consists of brief videotaped sequences in which various affective situations are enacted by a young woman. The subjects consisted of thirty LD and thirty NLD Caucasian boys between nine and twelve years of age.

Under attention-incentive conditions the findings indicated that the LD group did not obtain significantly lower accuracy scores than the NLD group on any of the PONS scales. However, the LD children were rated as more withdrawn, as reflected in higher scores on the Personality Problem scale of the BPC, relative to NLD children, and as less socially skilled. While not related to LD-NLD group differences, the PONS was related to intelligence and achievement scores, but not to measures of social competence when achievement was adequately controlled. Thus, these findings contrast with Bryan's in indicating that, under conditions designed to maximize attention, LD children performed equally to NLD children in comprehension of nonverbal communication. This suggests that attentional problems contributed to Bryan's findings.

The potential for combining social-relationship dimensions with behavior-problem dimensions to identify subgroups of learning disabled children at risk for specific outcomes is readily apparent. For example, childhood aggression has been associated with delinquency, as has poor childhood social adjustment as reflected in peer rejection measures (Roff 1972). Roff and Wirt (1984, 112) reasoned that "the conjunction of peer rejection and aggression should indicate significantly elevated risk for delinquency." Path analysis was used to assess the contribution of aggression in the context of peer rejection to the development of delinquency in a sample of 2,453 grade school children followed through record sources into young adulthood. Delinquency was defined as a formal juvenile court referral with most, but not all, being adjudicated. Peer status was determined by sociometric ratings by same-sex classmates. The results indicated that for males aggressive behavior in grade school in the context of peer rejection significantly correlated with delinquency. For low peer-status females, severity of family disturbances was the best single predictor of delinquency.

## Summary

The consideration of behavior problems in learning disabled children has moved from the view that learning problems reflected emotional problems, through categorical models that viewed school maladjustment either as a learning problem or as an emotional problem, to a model of secondary emotional problems resulting from the interaction of primary vulnerabilities and environmental stresses.

The factor structure of behavior problems in children with educational problems is very similar to that found in other normal and clinical groups of children: Conduct Disorder, Personality Problems, and Inadequacy-Immaturity. Children with learning disabilities demonstrate higher levels of these behavior problems than do control children but lower levels than children with primary behavior problems.

The evidence regarding the postulated link between learning disabilities and juvenile delinquency is conflictual. The conceptual models underlying the proposed link argue for a specificity of behavioral problems associated with learning disability. The basis or mechanism for the association of learning disability with juvenile delinquency needs to be elucidated. It can and should be pursued without negating that other behavior problem patterns are also demonstrated by children with learning disabilities.

Subgroup formation among children with learning disabilities on the basis of behavioral dimensions (such as aggression or hyperactivity) and cognitive dimensions affords an opportunity for increased specificity of intervention efforts. Adding social-relationship dimensions to the behavioral and cognitive dimensions offers the potential for identifying subgroups of learning disabled children who are at risk for specific outcomes.

# CHAPTER 6

# Synopsis of the Duke University Research Series

In conjunction with the evolving concept of developmental disabilities and advances in empirical delineation of childhood behavior problems, we have been involved in a series of related studies conducted in several clinics of Duke University Medical Center. Delineating the nature and extent of behavioral problems demonstrated by children with the chronic handicapping condition of developmental disabilities has been one of the goals of our research efforts. A simultaneous goal has been to contribute to the efforts to derive standardized, objective, and reliable methods for investigating and classifying behavioral disorders. Commensurate with the evolving concept of developmental disabilities, our approach differs from that of others in that we have focused upon the developmentally disabled as a group and have not focused upon specific subgroups formed on the basis of diagnostic conditions, such as mental retardation or autism. The subgroups of developmentally disabled that we have investigated have been formed on the basis of functional impairment. To date, we have conducted a total of nine studies, which will be summarized briefly. The approach we have taken has involved the utilization of the Missouri Children's Behavior Checklist (MCBC).

## Study I

Our initial effort was to determine whether children seen in two separate clinics for the developmentally disabled differed from each other on the dimensions of the MCBC and whether developmentally disabled children differed from nonreferred normal children (Thompson, Curry, and Yancy 1979). MCBC parental ratings were obtained at the time of intake on sixty-six males and fifteen females referred to the Georgetown University Affiliated Program for Child Development (GEO) and sixty males and thirty-two females referred to the Duke University Developmental Evaluation Center (DEC). The nonreferred controls consisted of twenty males and fifty-one females who had received routine physical exams in a pediatrician's office in Durham, North Carolina. The subjects ranged in age from two to fourteen years, and there were no significant differences in age among the groups.

The means and standard deviations of mother's behavior-checklist rating of GEO, DEC, and control males and females are

TABLE 1. Mean and Standard Deviation (SD) of Mothers' MCBC Ratings of Georgetown, Duke DEC, and Control Males and Females

| Scale | Males | | | Females | | |
|---|---|---|---|---|---|---|
| | GEO<br>($N = 66$) | DEC<br>($N = 60$) | Controls<br>($N = 27$) | GEO<br>($N = 15$) | DEC<br>($N = 32$) | Controls<br>($N = 31$) |
| Aggression | | | | | | |
| Mean | 7.80 | 5.70 | 3.22 | 6.80 | 5.28 | 4.03 |
| SD | 4.51 | 4.23 | 3.06 | 4.40 | 4.29 | 2.63 |
| Inhibition | | | | | | |
| Mean | 4.70 | 5.23 | 2.74 | 5.20 | 4.97 | 3.42 |
| SD | 2.76 | 2.64 | 1.70 | 3.00 | 2.67 | 2.54 |
| Activity level | | | | | | |
| Mean | 5.71 | 5.12 | 2.26 | 5.20 | 4.50 | 2.58 |
| SD | 2.70 | 2.59 | 2.03 | 3.38 | 2.62 | 1.65 |
| Sleep disturbance | | | | | | |
| Mean | 2.02 | 1.82 | 1.56 | 1.47 | 2.09 | 1.74 |
| SD | 2.02 | 1.99 | 1.74 | 1.25 | 2.04 | 1.48 |
| Somatization | | | | | | |
| Mean | 1.95 | 1.98 | 1.00 | 2.60 | 1.88 | 1.32 |
| SD | 1.79 | 1.63 | 1.27 | 1.68 | 1.77 | 1.19 |
| Sociability | | | | | | |
| Mean | 6.56 | 6.05 | 6.85 | 6.87 | 5.78 | 7.81 |
| SD | 2.14 | 2.10 | 2.21 | 2.45 | 1.98 | 1.54 |

presented in table 1 and depicted in figures 1 and 2. There were
no significant differences in mother's ratings of males or females
on any of the MCBC scales between the developmentally disabled children seen in the Georgetown and Duke Clinics. Thus,
the two samples were combined by sex. The MCBC results for
the combined Georgetown and Duke developmentally disabled
children were contrasted with those for the control children.
Developmentally disabled males and females were rated signifi-

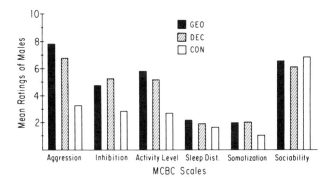

Fig. 1. Mothers' MCBC ratings of male children referred to the
Georgetown and Duke developmental disabilities clinics and
controls

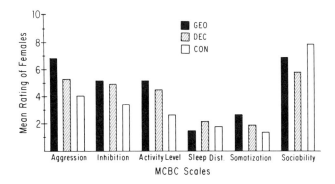

Fig. 2. Mothers' MCBC ratings of female children referred to the
Georgetown and Duke developmental disabilities clinics and
controls

cantly ($p < .05$) higher in Aggression, Inhibition, Activity Level, and Somatization than were the control males and females. Developmentally disabled females were also rated significantly lower on Sociability than were control females.

Several findings from the study were of interest. First, the homogeneity of the behavior ratings of the two groups of developmentally disabled males and females seen in different centers was striking. Second, the dimensions of behavior measured by the MCBC differentiated the developmentally disabled children from the normal controls. The next step was to determine whether the MCBC could discriminate between subgroups of referred children differing in presumed etiology and presumed severity of behavior disorder.

## Study II

Children referred to developmental disabilities clinics are suspected of having primary medical, developmental, or handicapping problems. Emotional or behavioral problems, if present, are presumed secondary to, or additional to, these developmental problems. On the other hand, children referred to psychiatric clinics are suspected of having primary emotional or behavioral problems. In Study II (Curry and Thompson 1979), it was hypothesized that children referred to a psychiatric clinic would be rated higher on the behavioral problem scales than children referred to a developmental disabilities clinic and that both clinic samples would be rated higher on these scales than nonreferred controls.

Subjects consisted of three samples of thirty males and twenty females obtained from the DEC, from the Community Guidance Clinic (CGC) (the outpatient psychiatric clinic of Duke Medical Center), and from children having routine physical examinations at several local pediatric clinics and offices. The subjects ranged in age from 2 to 12 with a mean of 7.46 years. The fifty subjects in each of these three samples were individually matched on sex, age, and socioeconomic status (SES).

The means and standard deviations of mothers' ratings of psychiatrically referred (CGC), developmentally disabled (DEC), and control children (CON) are presented in table 2 for males, females, and both sexes combined, and are depicted in figures 3, 4, and 5. Analysis of variance indicated a significant main effect for subject groups on all six scales ($p < .0001$). Main effects for sex were found on two scales: somatization ($p < .03$) and socialization ($p < .01$). Females were rated higher in somatic complaints and as more sociable than males. There were no significant interaction effects. Internal analysis of the main effects using the Duncan Multiple Range Test showed that children referred to the psychiatric clinic (CGC) were rated significantly higher in problems related to aggression, activity level, and sleep disturbance than were children referred to the developmental

TABLE 2.   Mean and Standard Deviation of Mothers' MCBC Ratings of Psychiatrically Referred, Developmentally Disabled, and Control Group Children

| Scale | Both Sexes | | | Males | | | Females | | |
|---|---|---|---|---|---|---|---|---|---|
| | CGC | DEC | CON | CGC | DEC | CON | CGC | DEC | CON |
| Aggression | | | | | | | | | |
| Mean | 8.18[a] | 6.02[b] | 3.50[c] | 8.27[a] | 6.60[a] | 3.93[b] | 8.05[a] | 5.15[b] | 2.85[b] |
| SD | 5.01 | 4.46 | 3.46 | 5.18 | 4.44 | 4.03 | 4.86 | 4.48 | 2.32 |
| Inhibition | | | | | | | | | |
| Mean | 5.22[a] | 4.92[a] | 2.48[b] | 4.93[a] | 4.67[a] | 2.53[b] | 5.65[a] | 5.30[a] | 2.40[b] |
| SD | 3.12 | 2.86 | 1.91 | 2.48 | 3.08 | 1.98 | 3.92 | 2.53 | 1.85 |
| Activity level | | | | | | | | | |
| Mean | 5.60[a] | 4.12[b] | 2.54[c] | 5.67[a] | 3.87[b] | 2.47[c] | 5.50[a] | 4.50[a] | 2.65[b] |
| SD | 2.68 | 2.42 | 1.94 | 2.49 | 2.36 | 1.96 | 3.00 | 2.52 | 1.95 |
| Sleep disturbance | | | | | | | | | |
| Mean | 3.28[a] | 2.14[b] | 1.20[c] | 3.43[a] | 1.60[b] | 1.23[b] | 3.05[a] | 2.95[a] | 1.15[b] |
| SD | 2.54 | 1.78 | 1.38 | 2.28 | 1.57 | 1.57 | 2.74 | 1.82 | 1.09 |
| Somatization | | | | | | | | | |
| Mean | 2.86[a] | 1.72[b] | 1.18[b] | 2.60[a] | 1.40[b] | 1.07[b] | 3.25[a] | 2.20[a,b] | 1.35[b] |
| SD | 1.99 | 1.69 | 1.06 | 1.99 | 1.49 | 1.10 | 1.97 | 1.88 | 0.98 |
| Sociability | | | | | | | | | |
| Mean | 6.80[a] | 5.70[b] | 6.72[a] | 6.37[a] | 5.53[a] | 6.23[a] | 7.45[a] | 5.95[b] | 7.45[a] |
| SD | 2.39 | 2.00 | 2.20 | 2.51 | 1.99 | 3.42 | 2.11 | 2.04 | 1.64 |

[a,b,c] Using the Duncan Multiple Range Test, means with the same superscript are not significantly different at $p < .05$.

disabilities clinic (DEC). Both clinical groups also were rated higher in these problem areas than were control children. The children referred to the psychiatric clinic were also rated as having significantly more somatic complaints than children referred to the DEC. The sociability scale did not discriminate between the psychiatric and control group children, but both groups were rated higher on sociability than the developmentally disabled children. Only the inhibition scale failed to discriminate between the two clinic groups, but both clinic groups were rated as significantly more inhibited than the control group.

Thus, the major hypotheses of this study were confirmed and the results provided additional support for the utility of the MCBC in reflecting dimensions of children's behavior that differentiate not only referred *from* nonreferred children but also *among* referred children. The results were also consistent with expectations regarding the extent of behavior problems in the children served in two different clinical settings.

The findings achieved in these first two studies were based on group differences in raw scores on one or more of the MCBC scales or dimensions. Further progress in developing adequate empirical methods for classification of children's behavior prob-

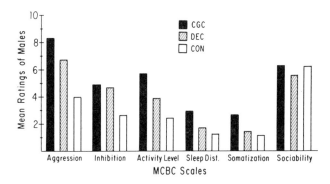

Fig. 3.   Mothers' MCBC ratings of male children referred to psychiatric and developmental disabilities clinics and nonreferred controls

lems would depend upon an ability for increased differentiation
in the samples of children studied. To increase the clinical utility
of the MCBC, it was necessary to cease relying solely upon global
group differences along single scales or dimensions and to develop a method of pattern identification and analysis based on
constellations or profiles of several dimensions.

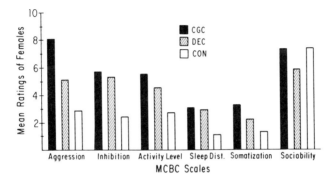

Fig. 4.   Mothers' MCBC ratings of female children referred to
psychiatric and developmental disabilities clinics and nonreferred
controls

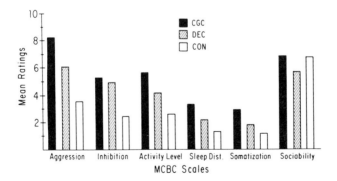

Fig. 5.   Mothers' MCBC ratings of children referred to psychiatric and developmental disabilities clinics and nonreferred
controls

## Study III

The purpose of Study III was to extend our previous work in identifying clinically relevant dimensions of behavior problems among developmentally disabled children. Cluster analysis of the MCBC was used to differentiate subgroups of children within the developmentally disabled population on the basis of patterns of behavioral problems (Curry and Thompson 1982). This pattern analysis provides information with respect to the prevalence of broad-band syndromes such as the Externalizing and Internalizing, and narrow-band syndromes such as Somatic Complaints and Sleep Disturbance. It also had been unclear whether elevated group means across scales are attributable to generalized mild to moderate levels of behavioral disturbance in most children with developmental disabilities or to a small subgroup with high levels of behavioral disturbance. Finally, pattern analysis based on empirically derived clusters would provide information regarding whether differences between the developmentally disabled and other populations are a function of different behavior patterns being demonstrated by different subgroups or are a function of different frequencies of the same behavior patterns.

Study III was conducted in two phases. A total of 257 children between two and twelve years of age referred to the DEC constituted the subjects for Phase I. These children were divided into two subsamples; sample A consisted of 89 males and 42 females and sample B consisted of 85 males and 41 females. There were no significant differences between the two subsamples in sex proportion, age, or SES.

Children's scores on the six MCBC scales were analyzed by hierarchical cluster analysis (Johnson 1967), and yielded four behavior profiles that could be replicated across both samples. These cluster profiles were: Aggressive-Active, Inhibited, Mixed Disturbance, and Normal. The behavior profiles in terms of mean MCBC scale scores in relation to normalized Z scores using norms derived from the normal control group described previously (Curry and Thompson 1979) are depicted in figures 6,

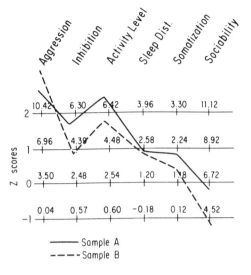

Fig. 6.   The MCBC Aggressive-Active behavior profile

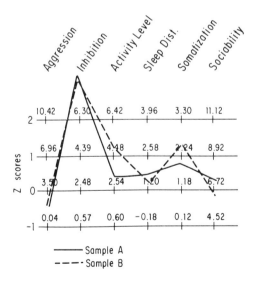

Fig. 7.   The MCBC Inhibited behavior profile

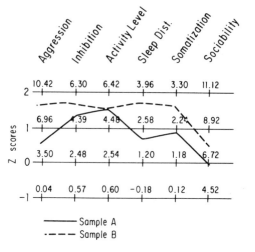

Fig. 8.  The MCBC Mixed disturbance profile

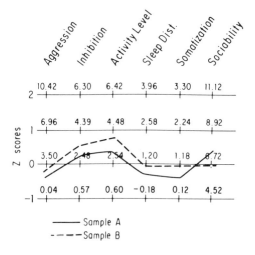

Fig. 9.  The MCBC Normal behavior profile

7, 8, and 9. A total of 74 percent and 78 percent of the two DEC samples could be classified into one of these four cluster profiles. Membership in one of the four clusters could not be predicted on the basis of age or sex.

The second phase of Study III was designed to determine whether the same types of clusters occurred in normal and psychiatrically referred children, and if so, whether the frequency distribution differed significantly among these groups. The subjects for this phase were 40 children taken from the sample of 50 nonreferred children described in Study II, and 105 children referred to the CGC. No significant differences existed among these samples in age or sex proportion.

The results are presented in table 3 and depicted in figure 10. A chi-square test of the differences in frequency distribution between the control and DEC samples was statistically significant ($p < .05$). There were proportionately fewer behavior-problem profiles and more Normal profiles in the nonreferred than in the DEC group. There were also proportionately fewer unclassified subjects in the nonreferred sample. The difference in frequency distribution between the DEC and CGC samples was also statistically significant ($p < .001$). There were proportionately more Agressive-Active and fewer Inhibited, Mixed, and Normal profiles in the psychiatrically referred sample (CGC) compared to the DEC sample. There was also a much higher percentage of unclassified cases in the CGC sample, suggesting that the cluster structure of the population of children seen in the psychiatric clinic probably contained profile subgroups that do

TABLE 3.  Frequency of MCBC Behavior Profile Membership by Nonreferred, Developmentally Disabled, and Psychiatrically Referred Children

| Behavior Profile | Nonreferred ($N = 40$) | DEC ($N = 257$) | CGC ($N = 105$) |
|---|---|---|---|
| Aggressive-Active | 1   (2.5%) | 22  (8%) | 19 (18%) |
| Inhibited | 2   (5) | 26 (10) | 4   (4) |
| Mixed | 5 (12.5) | 46 (18) | 13 (12) |
| Normal | 28 (70) | 101 (39) | 13 (12) |
| Unclassified | 4 (10) | 62 (24) | 56 (54) |

not occur in the developmentally disabled population and that
could be subsequently derived and identified.

This study yielded several useful findings. First, four behavior
profiles were identified and replicated. Second, the behavior
profiles identified suggest that the behavioral problems in children with developmental disabilities can follow the broad-band
pattern of Externalizers (Aggressive-Active) and Internalizers
(Inhibition). In addition, a relatively undifferentiated pattern of
disturbance was evident (Mixed). Third, the frequency of occurrence of behavior profiles differed across clinical and nonreferred samples. Fourth, the use of behavior-problem profiles in
this study enables possible clarification of findings of previous
studies.

The previous finding that, as a group, the developmentally
disabled children demonstrated more behavioral problems than
the controls but less than children referred to the child psychiatric clinic appeared to be attributable to the relatively small
proportion of developmentally disabled children showing behavior disorders. The present results do not suggest that a generalized mild level of disturbance is characteristic of most developmentally disabled children.

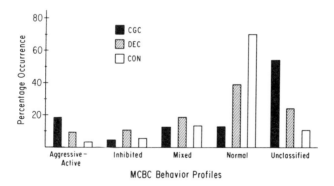

Fig. 10.   Percentage occurrence of MCBC behavior profiles in
children referred to psychiatric and developmental disabilities
clinics and nonreferred controls

When profile rules obtained from the DEC cluster analysis were applied to the CGC patients, the frequency distribution of cases was markedly different. However, only the Aggressive-Active children were more numerous in the CGC sample than in the DEC sample. The other types of disturbances were proportionately more rare in the CGC sample, and the proportion of unclassified cases was much higher. Taken together, these findings suggest that the differences between DEC and CGC samples are not simply a matter of frequency of occurrence of behavior patterns. There are likely to be different types of behavior patterns in the CGC sample. Additional profiles would need to be derived in the group of psychiatrically referred children in order to classify and understand that population more adequately.

## Study IV

Given the findings of these early studies, the MCBC appeared to have potential utility as a basis for the formation of clinically relevant subgroups of children. The next required step was to prove the construct validity of the various MCBC scales and profiles in terms of their ability to reflect the specific behavior dimensions that they proport to tap and their ability to reflect specific clinical manifestations that differentiate subgroups of children. The goal of the next study was to provide construct validity information by investigating the relationship between MCBC scales and behavior profiles, demographic factors, clinical findings, and recommendations for developmentally disabled children (Thompson and Curry 1983).

This study used the data base from the 301 children seen for an interdisciplinary evaluation at the DEC that was described previously (see Chap. 3). The sample consisted of 217 children between two and thirteen years of age for whom MCBC data were available. Subgroups of children were formed on the basis of demographic factors and the presence or absence of diagnoses, specific clinical findings, and recommendations recorded in their charts. The demographic factors included sex, race, and SES. Diagnoses included mental retardation, learning disabili-

ties, and a general category of physical/somatic findings. Specific
clinical findings included the behavioral problems of overly aggressive, overly active, and attentional deficit. While not directly
corresponding to any MCBC scale profiles, several subgroups
were formed on the basis of presence or absence of affective
problems, such as sad/withdrawn, anxious/fearful, and low self-
concept. Finally, subgroups were formed on the basis of presence
or absence of a specific recommendation of child therapy and
parent therapy. Information regarding the construct validity of
the MCBC was obtained by contrasting MCBC scales and behavioral profiles demonstrated by the subgroups formed on the basis
of the presence or absence of these specific clinical findings.

There were few significant differences in MCBC scale means
as a function of the demographic factors of sex, race, and SES.
Males were rated higher on the aggression scale than females
(5.45 versus 3.84, $p < .01$). Caucasians had significantly higher
ratings on the sleep disturbance scale than black children (1.86
versus 1.22, $p < .01$), and those in the bottom two SES levels were
rated significantly higher on activity level (4.80 versus 4.03, $p <
.05$) and somatization (1.74 versus 1.12, $p < .05$) than those in the
top three SES levels. There were no significant differences in the
percentage occurrence of any of the MCBC behavioral profiles
as a function of these demographic factors.

There was only one significant difference in MCBC scale
means as a function of the presence or absence of major diagnostic categories. Diagnosis represented an integration of medical,
neuromotor, cognitive, psychosocial, language, and educational
findings. Those diagnosed as mentally retarded were rated significantly higher in activity level (5.38 versus 4.51, $p < .05$) than
those without this diagnosis. There were no significant differences in percentage occurrence of behavioral profiles as a
function of the presence or absence of learning disability or
mental retardation. (For a diagnosis of mental retardation, it was
necessary to have a Bayley MDI or a WISC-R—Full Scale IQ of
69 or a Stanford Binet IQ of 67. The definition of learning

disabilities was that provided in the *Federal Register*, 41(250) 65083, December 29, 1977).

There were no significant differences in the scale means or in percentage of occurrence of behavioral profiles as a function of the presence or absence of the findings of physical or somatic problems. Of particular interest is the absence of any significant difference on the somatization scale, suggesting that the ratings on this scale are not reflecting problems of a truly physical nature.

In contrast to the few significant differences in MCBC scales and profiles demonstrated as a function of demographic factors or broad diagnostic categories, the relationship between the MCBC and behavior problems identified by the interdisciplinary team was relatively strong. Those children found to be overly aggressive were significantly higher on the aggression (8.09 versus 4.40, $p < .0001$), activity level (5.50 versus 4.42, $p < .01$), and somatization (2.19 versus 1.46, $p < .01$) scales than those not found to be overly aggressive. In addition, the percentage of occurrence of behavioral profiles differed significantly with 28.3 percent of those found to be overly aggressive demonstrating the Aggressive-Active behavior profile compared to only 3.7 percent of those without this finding ($p < .0001$). Children found to be overly active were rated significantly higher on the activity level scale (6.12 versus 4.52, $p < .01$) and had a significantly higher occurrence of the Aggressive-Active behavior profile (25 percent versus 6 percent, $p < .05$) than those without this finding. Children with attentional deficit problems were rated significantly higher on the aggression (6.21 versus 4.68, $p < .05$), activity level (5.92 versus 4.30, $p < .0001$), and sociability (7.16 versus 6.37, $p < .09$) scales, but were not significantly different in the percentage of occurrence of behavioral profiles than those children without the finding of attentional deficit. The finding of attentional deficit represented a combination of the findings of poor attention span and distractibility recorded in the child's clinic record.

The relationship of the MCBC with the findings of affective

problems was not as strong as the relationship of the MCBC with behavior problems. Those with the finding of sad/withdrawn or anxious/fearful or low self-concept each were rated significantly higher on the somatization scale than those without these findings (respectively: 1.96 versus 1.43, $p < .05$; 2.08 versus 1.75, $p < .01$; 1.98 versus 1.44, $p < .05$). In addition, those found to have a low self-concept had a significantly higher percentage of occurrence of the Inhibited behavior profile (18.52 percent) than those without this finding (7.98 percent). Those found to be anxious/fearful had a significantly ($p < .05$) smaller percentage occurrence of the Normal behavior profile (22.45 percent) than those without this finding (40.48 percent). There were no significant differences in percentage occurrence of any of the behavior profiles on the basis of presence or absence of the findings of sad/withdrawn.

Subgroups were also formed on the basis of recommendations. The children for whom therapy was recommended differed significantly from those for whom the recommendation was not made only in terms of a higher rating on the somatization scale (1.86 versus 1.37, $p < .05$). Children for whom recommendations for parent therapy or counseling were made were rated significantly higher on the aggression scale (5.67 versus 4.24, $p < .01$) and sleep disturbance scale (1.97 versus 1.33, $p < .05$) than those whose parents did not receive this recommendation. In addition, children of the parent-therapy subgroup demonstrated a significantly higher occurrence of the Aggressive-Active behavior profile (11.21 percent versus 64 percent, $p < .05$) and a significantly lower percentage occurrence of the Normal behavior profile (29.91 percent versus 42.73 percent, $p < .05$) than did the subgroup of children for whom parent therapy was not recommended.

To obtain additional information about the construct validity of the MCBC behavior profiles, subgroups were formed on the basis of presence of each profile. The percentage occurrence of the various diagnoses, findings, and recommendations demonstrated by each behavior problem profile subgroup was compared to the percentage occurrence demonstrated by the Normal profile subgroup. The percentage occurrence of the behavior profiles was as follows: Aggressive-Active (7.37 percent); Inhibited (10.6 percent); Mixed (20.74 percent); Normal (36.41 percent); and 24.89 percent were unclassified.

In comparison with those with the Normal profile, those with the Aggressive-Active profile demonstrated significantly higher occurrences of the finding of overly aggressive (56.25 percent versus 11.39 percent, $p < .0001$) and the recommendation for parent therapy (75 percent versus 40.51 percent, $p < .01$). Those with the Inhibited profile demonstrated a significantly higher percentage of occurrence of the finding of low self-concept (43.48 percent versus 20.25 percent, $p < .01$). Those with an unclassified profile exhibited a significantly higher percentage of occurrences of attentional deficit (25.93 percent versus 12.66 percent, $p < .05$) and the recommendation of parent therapy (57.41 percent versus 40.51 percent, $p < .05$). The Mixed profile subgroup did not differ significantly from the Normal profile subgroup in percentage occurrence of any of the diagnoses, findings, or recommendations.

The construct validity of the MCBC scales and behavior profiles is substantially increased by this work. Of particular importance are the very few significant differences as a function of demographic factors and broad diagnostic categories, in conjunction with the significant differences among clinical finding subgroups on the particular MCBC scales and behavior profiles that are purported to measure these dimension. The relationship between the MCBC and behavior problems was relatively strong. The relationship of the MCBC with affective problems was less strong. Statistically significant differences were found on the somatization scale for those with versus those without specific affective findings, but differences in scale means were small and of little clinical utility, particularly with individual cases. The relationship between the MCBC and recommendations for therapy was ambiguous. For example, of those with a Normal behavior profile, 40 percent had a recommendation for parent therapy and 35 percent for child therapy. This is similar to the 26 percent false positive rate reported by Defilippis (1979). It is likely that a number of other factors, such as the quality and availability of support systems, in addition to the type and extent of behavior problems, are involved in clinical decisions regarding the recommendation of therapy.

The lack of any significant relationship between the Mixed behavior profile and clinical findings suggests that this pattern is not yet sufficiently differentiated. In addition, 25 percent of the sample yielded unclassified behavior profiles, and considered as a subgroup, they demonstrated significantly higher percentages of attentional deficit problems and recommendations for parent therapy than did the Normal profile subgroup. This finding suggests the potential for evolving additional behavior profiles for the developmentally disabled from within the now unclassified subgroup. It will be remembered from Study III that it was thought that additional behavior profiles could be derived from the psychiatric sample as well.

## Study V

Having demonstrated the utility of the MCBC scales and behavior profiles for differentiating among children referred to psychiatric and developmental disabilities clinics and nonreferred controls, the goal of the next study was to evaluate the MCBC as a method of early identification of behavioral problems. The context for this study was an effort at early identification of preschool children "at risk" for developmental and learning problems (Thompson et al. 1982). Two questions were formulated: (1) Do preschool children who are found to be "at risk" for developmental and learning problems receive different ratings on the MCBC scales and profiles than children not found to be "at risk"? (2) How do the MCBC results of the "at risk" and "nonrisk" preschool children compare with results demonstrated by preschool children seen in a clinic for developmental disabilities?

The subjects consisted of 105 children who were participants in a prekindergarten health-screening program in a rural county of North Carolina. There were 61 males and 44 females ranging from four and one-half to five and one-half years of age. This sample was divided into two subgroups based on their performance on the McCarthy Scales of Children's Abilities. Those obtaining a General Cognitive Index (GCI) < 84 were characterized "at risk." Those with a GCI > 84 were characterized as "nonrisk." There were 42 children at risk (28 males and 14 females; 18 Caucasians and 24 blacks) and 63 nonrisk (33 males, 30 females; 44 Caucasians, 19 blacks). The comparison sample of preschool developmentally disabled children was obtained from the data base of children seen at the DEC. There were 20 children in the sample who fell in the appropriate age range (14 males, 6 females; 11 Caucasians, 9 blacks). The DEC sample did not differ significantly from the screening sample in terms of race, sex, or SES.

TABLE 4.   Mean and Standard Deviation of MCBC Scale Ratings for Nonrisk, At Risk, and Developmentally Disabled Children

| Scale | Nonrisk ($N = 63$) | At Risk ($N = 42$) | DEC ($N = 20$) |
|---|---|---|---|
| Aggression | | | |
| Mean | 2.76 | 3.78 | 6.00 |
| SD | 2.41 | 3.69 | 4.40 |
| Inhibition | | | |
| Mean | 2.71 | 3.57 | 5.65 |
| SD | 1.74 | 2.35 | 2.35 |
| Activity level | | | |
| Mean | 2.56 | 3.67 | 4.70 |
| SD | 2.05 | 2.47 | 2.49 |
| Sleep disturbance | | | |
| Mean | 1.27 | 1.52 | 1.50 |
| SD | 1.52 | 1.71 | 1.32 |
| Somatization | | | |
| Mean | 0.89 | 1.02 | 1.10 |
| SD | 0.92 | 1.47 | 1.21 |
| Sociability | | | |
| Mean | 7.60 | 6.60 | 6.70 |
| SD | 1.72 | 2.00 | 2.49 |

The means and standard deviations of MCBC scale ratings for the nonrisk, at risk, and developmentally disabled children (DEC) are presented in table 4. MCBC scale means are depicted by group in figure 11. It can be seen in figure 11 that in general the at risk group fell between the DEC and nonrisk groups on the MCBC scales. A one-way multivariate analysis of variance comparing these means showed that the three groups differed significantly ($p < .001$) on the MCBC with significant univariate Fs obtained for the aggression, inhibition, activity level, and sociability scales. Duncan's range test was used to evaluate specific group differences ($p < .05$). The at risk children demonstrated significantly higher ratings on the inhibition and the activity level scales and lower ratings on the sociability scale than the nonrisk children. The developmentally disabled children were rated significantly higher on the aggression, inhibition, and activity level scales than the nonrisk children and significantly higher on the aggression and inhibition scales than the at risk children.

In terms of behavior profiles, it can be seen in table 5 that the percentages are ordered monotonically across the three groups with the DEC group exhibiting the most Aggressive-Active, Inhibited, Mixed, and unclassified profiles and the nonrisk group

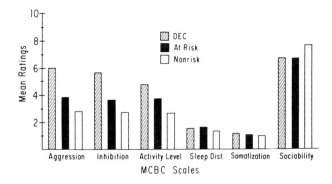

Fig. 11.   Mothers' MCBC ratings of developmentally disabled, at risk, and nonrisk preschool age children

the most Normal profiles. In each case, the at risk group percentages fall between the DEC and nonrisk groups. The three groups differed significantly on the percentages of Normal versus nonnormal profiles ($\chi^2$ (2) = 15.9, $p < .001$) and the percentages of unclassified versus classified profiles ($\chi^2$ (2) = 6.42, $p < .05$).

The differences in the percentages of Aggressive-Active profiles between the at risk and nonrisk groups and between the nonrisk and DEC groups approached significance (Fisher Exact Probabilities Test, $p < .06$). But there was no significant difference in percentage of occurrence between the at risk and DEC groups. There were no significant differences among the three groups in the percentage of Inhibited profiles nor Mixed profiles.

The results of Study V indicated that preschool children found during screening to be nonrisk or at risk for developmental and learning problems differ from each other and from developmentally disabled preschool children on several of the MCBC scales and behavior profiles. The at risk children clearly demonstrated fewer Normal profiles and received ratings on the other behavior-problem scales and profiles midway between those for the nonrisk and DEC preschool children. More importantly, differences between the at risk and nonrisk preschool children emerged on scales (activity level, inhibition, sociability) and behavior profiles (Aggressive-Active), reflective of the broadband Externalizing and Internalizing behavior problems of older children seen in psychiatric clinics.

The findings suggest that preschool children who are demon-

TABLE 5.  Percentage of MCBC Behavior Profiles Demonstrated by Nonrisk, At Risk, and Developmentally Disabled Children

| Behavior Profile | Nonrisk ($N = 63$) | At Risk ($N = 42$) | DEC ($N = 20$) |
|---|---|---|---|
| Aggressive-Inhibited | 10.0 | 7.1 | 0.0 |
| Inhibited | 15.0 | 9.5 | 3.2 |
| Mixed | 15.0 | 11.9 | 11.1 |
| Normal | 30.0 | 57.1 | 77.8 |
| Unclassified | 30.0 | 14.3 | 7.9 |

strating the potential for developmental and learning difficulties are also demonstrating the potential for behavior problems. This was the first time that the MCBC had been shown to differentiate between meaningful subgroups of nonreferred children. This study adds support to the interpretation of the MCBC differences as reflecting differences in children's behavior. Since both groups were nonreferred, the obtained differences could not have been related to differences in parents' willingness to acknowledge behavior problems as a function of whether they took their child to a pediatric or a psychiatric clinic.

Given the increased incidence of behavioral and psychological problems in children with chronic illness, delineating the etiology of these behavior problems has been of concern. In some instances, the developmental and behavioral problems can be understood as a consequence of earlier environmental factors or CNS (central nervous system) dysfunction. In other instances, the behavioral problems can be understood as the consequence of stress and frustration encountered in school by the child with developmental problems. Because most studies of learning and behavioral problems involve school-aged children, disentangling these effects has been difficult. However, in this study, the risk of behavior problems cannot be related to school experience. Rather, the risks for learning and behavior problems coexist and are related to an individual's level of developmental or cognitive functioning.

## Study VI

The next study was undertaken to continue the efforts to derive behavior problem profiles (Curry and Thompson 1985). It was hypothesized that additional and/or different behavior-problem profile subgroups could be delineated by extending the hierarchical cluster analysis technique to MCBC data obtained from children referred to a child psychiatry clinic (CGC). Subjects included in the first phase were 130 children between the ages of three and twelve years who had been referred to the CGC. The

subjects were split into two samples (A and B), which were
equated on average age, SES, and proportion of males to females. Hierarchical cluster analysis yielded seven clusters that
replicated across both samples A and B and are depicted in
figures 12 through 18. Two clusters reflected behavior problems
of an internalizing nature. The Inhibited-Nonaggressive cluster
is characterized by a relatively low score on aggression and a high
score on inhibition. The Low Social Skills cluster is characterized by a low score on socialization. Four clusters reflected
behavior problems of an externalizing nature. The Aggressive-
Inhibited cluster is characterized by elevation on both aggression
and inhibition. The Mildly Aggressive cluster is characterized by
an elevation on aggression with a marked absence of inhibition.
The Aggressive-Active cluster is characterized by elevations on
both aggression and activity level. The Undifferentiated cluster is
characterized by elevation on aggression, inhibition, activity
level, and somatization. The Behavior-Problem-Free cluster is
characterized by relatively low scores on all scales.

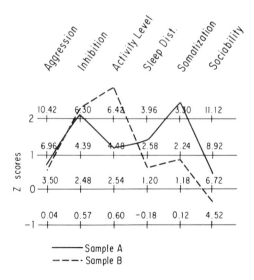

Fig. 12.   The MCBC Inhibited-Nonaggressive behavior profile

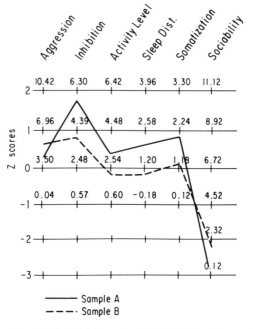

Fig. 13.   The MCBC Low Social Skills behavior profile

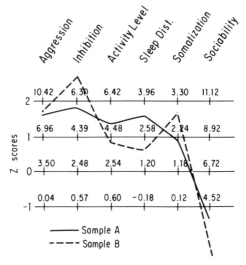

Fig. 14.   The MCBC Aggressive-Inhibited behavior profile

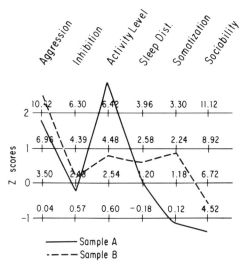

Fig. 15.   The MCBC Mildly Aggressive behavior profile

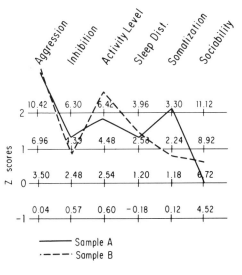

Fig. 16.   The MCBC Aggressive-Active behavior profile

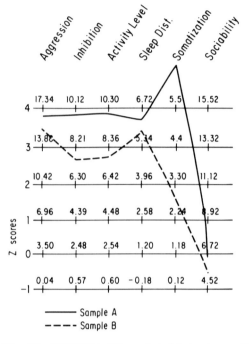

Fig. 17.  The MCBC Undifferentiated behavior profile

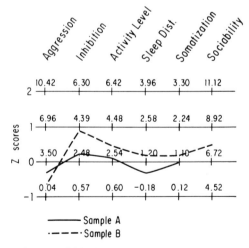

Fig. 18.  The MCBC Behavior-Problem-Free profile

The purpose of the second phase was to determine whether the same kinds of behavior-problem profiles occurred in the normal and developmentally disabled children and whether there were any differences in frequency distribution across the groups of children. Subjects in Phase II were 65 children between the ages of three and twelve years who had been referred to the DEC plus 44 nonreferred control children, in addition to the 130 children from the combined samples A and B from the CGC. Not only did the seven-cluster solution provide good coverage of the CGC samples (77 percent and 75 percent) but it also classified 74 percent of the children in the developmental disabilities sample. It will be remembered that the original four-cluster solution classified 74 percent and 78 percent, respectively, of two samples of developmentally disabled children, but only 46 percent of the child psychiatry sample. Table 6 depicts the significantly different ($p < .05$) frequency distributions of the seven clusters for the three samples. In general, the CGC children, compared to the DEC children, show fewer internalizing problems (Inhibited-Nonaggressive and Low Social Skills) and more externalizing problems (Mildly Aggressive; Aggressive-Active; Aggressive-Inhibited; and Undifferentiated). Most nonreferred

TABLE 6.    Frequency of MCBC Behavior Profiles Demonstrated by Psychiatrically Referred, Developmentally Disabled, and Nonreferred Children

| Profile | CGC ($N = 130$) | DEC ($N = 65$) | CON ($N = 44$) |
|---|---|---|---|
| Behavior Problem Profiles | 86 (66%) | 38 (58%) | 13 (30%) |
|   Internalizing | 28 (22) | 25 (38) | 10 (23) |
|     Inhibited-Nonaggressive | 21 (16) | 19 (29) | 6 (14) |
|     Low Social Skills | 7 (5) | 6 (9) | 4 (9) |
|   Externalizing | 58 (45) | 13 (29) | 3 (7) |
|     Aggressive-Inhibited | 14 (11) | 3 (5) | 0 (0) |
|     Mildly Aggressive | 22 (17) | 4 (6) | 2 (3) |
|     Aggressive-Active | 18 (14) | 6 (9) | 1 (1) |
|     Undifferentiated | 4 (3) | 0 (0) | 0 (0) |
| Behavior-Problem Free | 13 (10) | 10 (15) | 24 (54) |
| Unclassified | 31 (24) | 17 (26) | 7 (11) |

children demonstrating any type of behavior disturbances had either the Inhibited-Nonaggressive profile or the Low Social Skills profile, and 54 percent had the Behavior-Problem-Free profile versus 10 percent for the CGC children and 15 percent for the DEC children.

The seven-cluster solution derived from a child psychiatry sample was a more effective classification system than the four-cluster solution previously derived with developmentally disabled children. The seven-cluster solution provided more refined subgroups of behavior-problem profile patterns, particularly of aggression and inhibition, than the four-cluster solution, and it provided equally good coverage for children referred to a child psychiatry clinic and to a clinic for the developmentally disabled.

## Study VII

The next step was to begin to provide information about the construct validity of the seven behavior profile clusters (Thompson and Curry 1985). We again utilized the DEC data base that was described previously and that was also used for the construct validity study of the original four behavior profile clusters. The MCBC data were analyzed to determine the relationship between the seven clusters and both the clinical findings and recommendations that stemmed from the interdisciplinary evaluation of a sample of 217 children seen at the DEC. The seven-cluster solution classified 73 percent of the 217 children with the frequencies depicted in table 7. Similar to the four-cluster solution, there were almost no significant differences in percentage of occurrence of any of the seven behavior profiles as a function of demographic factors or broad diagnostic categories of learning disability or mental retardation. There were significant differences as a function of subgroups formed on the basis of presence or absence of clinical findings of behavior problems. For example, of those found to be overly aggressive, 19 percent demonstrated the Aggressive-Active profile versus 3 percent of those without this finding ($p < .002$). Of those found to have an

attentional deficit versus those without this finding, there was a
significantly higher percentage of occurrence of the Mildly Aggressive profile (13 percent versus 4.5 percent; $p < .06$) and a
significantly lower percentage of occurrence of the Inhibited-
Nonaggressive profile (18 percent versus 34 percent; $p < .05$), and
none demonstrated the Low Social Skills profile (0 versus 8
percent; $p < .05$).

Additional construct validity support was provided for two of
the behavior-problem profiles by comparing the frequencies of
occurrence of clinical findings and recommendations between
subgroups demonstrating each behavior-problem profile and the
Behavior-Problem-Free Profile. Those with the Aggressive-
Active profile demonstrated a significantly higher percentage
occurrence of the overly aggressive finding (55 percent versus 15
percent; $p < .01$) and the recommendation for child therapy (64
percent versus 31 percent; $p < .05$) and parent therapy (91
percent versus 42 percent; $p < .003$). Those with the Aggressive-
Inhibited profile demonstrated a significantly higher percentage
occurrence of the recommendation for child therapy (80 percent
versus 31 percent; $p < .05$).

It needs to be stressed that the reanalysis of the previous data

TABLE 7.   Frequency of MCBC Behavior Profiles
Demonstrated by Developmentally Disabled
Children

| Profile | DEC ($N = 217$) |
|---|---|
| Behavior Problem Profiles | 111 (51%) |
|   Internalizing | 82 (38) |
|     Inhibited-Nonaggressive | 67 (31) |
|     Low Social Skills | 15 (7) |
|   Externalizing | 29 (13) |
|     Aggressive-Inhibited | 5 (2) |
|     Mildly Aggressive | 13 (6) |
|     Aggressive-Active | 11 (6) |
|     Undifferentiated | 0 (0) |
| Behavior-Problem Free | 48 (22) |
| Unclassified | 58 (27) |

base using the new seven-cluster solution represents just the beginning of the necessary construct validity assessment. Additional studies with multiple samples of children referred to clinical settings are required, in which the association of profiles and diagnoses, recommendations for therapy, and therapy outcome can be determined.

## Study VIII

This chapter has shown that seven behavior-profile subgroups had been developed that classified approximately 75 percent of children seen in clinics for developmental disabilities and in psychiatric clinics. It was subsequently decided to reanalyze the data from the at risk study (Study V) to determine what else might be revealed about the behavior problems of children at risk for developmental problems by using a more extensive and delineated system. The MCBC ratings of forty-two at risk (GCI < 84), sixty-three nonrisk (GCI > 84), and twenty developmentally disabled preschool children were reanalyzed to determine the frequency of occurrence of the seven behavior profiles. The findings are depicted in table 8.

TABLE 8.  Frequency of MCBC Behavior Profiles Demonstrated by Developmentally Disabled, At Risk, and Nonrisk Children

| Profile | DEC ($N = 20$) | At Risk ($N = 42$) | Nonrisk ($N = 63$) | $\chi^2$ $p <$ |
|---|---|---|---|---|
| Behavior Problem Profiles | 11 (55%) | 22 (52%) | 12 (19%) | .0001 |
| Internalizing | 11 (55) | 19 (45) | 7 (11) | .001 |
| Inhibited-Nonaggressive | 9 (45) | 15 (36) | 7 (11) | .001 |
| Low Social Skills | 2 (10) | 4 (10) | 0 (0) | .04 |
| Externalizing | 0 (0) | 3 (7) | 5 (8) | NS |
| Aggressive-Inhibited | 0 (0) | 0 (0) | 0 (0) | NS |
| Mildly Aggressive | 0 (0) | 0 (0) | 4 (6) | NS |
| Aggressive-Active | 0 (0) | 3 (7) | 1 (2) | NS |
| Undifferentiated | 0 (0) | 0 (0) | 0 (0) | NS |
| Behavior-Problem Free | 1 (5) | 12 (29) | 46 (73) | .0001 |
| Unclassified | 8 (40) | 8 (19) | 5 (8) | .003 |

The seven-profile solution was able to classify 81 percent of the at risk, 97 percent of the nonrisk, and 60 percent of the DEC samples. It can be seen that there were a number of significant differences in percentage occurrence of various behavior profiles across the three groups. The highest percentage occurrence of behavior-problem profiles was demonstrated by the DEC group (55 percent), followed by the at risk group (52 percent) and nonrisk group (19 percent) ($p < .0001$). Correspondingly, the highest percentage occurrence of Behavior-Problem-Free profiles occurred in the nonrisk group (73 percent), followed by the at risk group (29 percent) and the DEC group (5 percent) ($p < .0001$). It can also be seen that the preponderance of behavior-problem profiles were of the internalizing type, the majority being the Inhibited-Nonaggressive profile. The same relative relationship among the groups is evident with the highest percentage occurrence in the DEC group, followed by the at risk and nonrisk subgroups.

In comparison with the four-cluster solution, the seven-cluster solution still enables us to see that the preschoolers who are at risk for learning problems also demonstrate behavior problems above those of nonrisk children and approaching those of developmentally disabled preschoolers. Furthermore, the impact of the more refined delineation of the seven-cluster solution is made apparent by comparing the Behavior-Problem-Free profiles with the Normal profile of the four-cluster solution. The percentage occurrence is similar for the nonrisk group—73 percent Behavior-Problem-Free versus 78 percent Normal. However, in the DEC group, while 30 percent demonstrated the Normal profile, this was reduced to 5 percent demonstrating the Behavior-Problem-Free profile. For the at risk group, the reduction was from 57 percent to 7 percent. Whereas the four-cluster solution resulted in no Aggressive profiles for the nonrisk, 10 percent for the DEC, and 7 percent for the at risk groups, the seven-cluster solution yielded 8 percent, 0 percent, and 7 percent, respectively.

While there were no significant differences among groups in the percentage occurrence of the Inhibited profile of the four-cluster solution, significant group differences were demonstrated for the Inhibited-Nonaggressive profile ($p < .001$) and for the Low Social Skills profile ($p < .04$) of the seven-cluster solution. We are struck again by the occurrence of the internalizing type behavior-problem profiles with children who have, or who are at risk for, developmental and learning problems.

## Study IX

As noted previously, a persistent question has been the type and extent of behavior problems demonstrated by children with educational problems. Another question has been whether the type and extent of behavior problems differ among subgroups of children with education problems such as those with learning disabilities or mental retardation. The review of literature presented previously indicates that children with educational problems as a group demonstrate more behavioral problems than control children but fewer than children with emotional problems. Differences in behavior problems among subgroups of educational problems have been inconsistently reported.

The purpose of the next study was to assess the types and extent of behavior problems demonstrated by a particular group of children seen at the DEC: children with poor school performance. Furthermore, subgroups of these children with poor school performance were formed to enable comparisons of type and extent of behavior problems. The subgroups were comprised of children with learning disabilities, mental retardation, and borderline intellectual functioning, as well as those not learning disabled, borderline, nor mentally retarded. The initial focus was on the subgroup of children with poor school performance who were considered to be learning disabled.

To accomplish this task a prospective study was undertaken at the DEC. Starting in July 1982, a research protocol was established for all school-age children (six to seventeen years of age) seen at the DEC. The children received an individually administered intelligence test (WISC-R) and the Woodcock Johnson

Psychoeducational Battery—Tests of Achievement. Their parents (most frequently mother) completed the MCBC. The protocol was continued for two years until June of 1984.[1]

During the two-year time period intellectual, achievement, and MCBC data were obtained on 79 children. There were 55 (70 percent) males and 24 (30 percent) females and 48 (61 percent) Caucasian, 28 (35 percent) black, and 3 (4 percent) other races. The age range was from 6.9 years to 15.1 years with a mean of 10.1 years.

The difficulty in conceptually and operationally defining learning disabilities has been legend. In this study, the classification of a child as having a learning disability was operationally based on the concept of average-or-above intellectual functioning with a substantial deficit in academic functioning. Three performance criteria were established in the protocol to classify individual children with poor school performance as learning disabled. First, the teacher and/or the parent reported a serious learning problem. Second, the child was found to have at least average intelligence as measured by the WISC-R. Average intelligence was defined as Verbal Scale IQ $\geq$ 85 or Performance Scale IQ $\geq$ 85 or Full Scale IQ $\geq$ 85. Third, there was a deficit in academic achievement as determined by Woodcock Johnson test scores less than or equal to the twentieth percentile on the reading or math or written language or knowledge clusters. Each child was classified as learning disabled or not learning disabled.

Using these criteria, 34 (43 percent) of the 79 children seen over a two-year period were classified as learning disabled and 45 (57 percent) were classified as not learning disabled. Of the 34 learning disabled, 26 (76 percent) were males and 8 (24 percent) were females. Of the 45 not learning disabled, 29 (64 percent) were males and 16 (36 percent) were females.

Analysis of the intellectual and achievement test results of the children classified as learning disabled and those classified as not

[1]The assistance of Louise Lampron and Debra Johnson is gratefully acknowledged.

learning disabled are depicted in table 9. Since a substantial deficit ($\leq$ twentieth percentile) in achievement was one of the criteria to define the LD group, it is to be expected that there would be significant differences in achievment test score means (t-test for independent samples) between the LD and non-LD groups. It is interesting to note that only one significant difference between groups occurred in intelligence. The LD group had a significantly higher ($p < .04$) Performance Scale IQ.

The means and standard deviations of the LD and non-LD groups on each of the MCBC scales are presented in table 10. There were no significant differences in means (t-test for independent samples) between the LD and non-LD groups on any of the MCBC scales.

Table 11 depicts the findings regarding MCBC Behavior Profiles demonstrated by the LD and non-LD groups. The Behavior Problem Profile category reflects the total number of Behavior-Problem Profiles (Inhibited-Nonaggressive; Low Social Skills; Aggressive-Inhibited; Mildly Aggressive; Aggressive-Active; Undifferentiated) demonstrated by each group. It can be seen that

TABLE 9.   Mean and Standard Deviation of Intellectual and Achievement Test Scores for Learning Disabled and Non–Learning Disabled Children Seen in a Developmental Disabilities Center

| Measure | LD (N = 34) | | Non-LD (N = 45) | | |
| | Mean | SD | Mean | SD | p < |
| --- | --- | --- | --- | --- | --- |
| WISC-R | | | | | |
| Verbal Scale IQ | 85.8 | 12.0 | 85.4 | 20.0 | NS |
| Performance Scale IQ | 90.5 | 9.8 | 83.0 | 19.9 | .04 |
| Full Scale IQ | 87.2 | 8.6 | 83.4 | 20.1 | NS |
| Woodcock Johnson Psycho-educational Battery[a] | | | | | |
| Reading cluster | 17.5 | 16.4 | 33.6 | 34.7 | .02 |
| Math cluster | 15.9 | 15.6 | 28.5 | 32.5 | .04 |
| Written language cluster | 15.9 | 16.9 | 32.7 | 32.1 | .007 |
| Knowledge cluster | 23.5 | 22.0 | 32.1 | 35.6 | NS |

[a]Percentile scores for age

59 percent of the LD group and 69 percent of the non-LD group demonstrated a Behavior-Problem Profile, while 6 percent of the LD group and 7 percent of the non-LD group demonstrated the Behavior-Problem-Free profile. The unclassified category constituted 35 percent of the LD group and 24 percent of the non-LD group. There was no significant difference in the occurrence of these three categories of MCBC profiles between the LD and non-LD groups as determined by chi square. In terms of each

TABLE 10.  Mean and Standard Deviation of MCBC Scale Ratings for Learning Disabled and Non–Learning Disabled Children Seen in a Developmental Disabilities Center

|  | LD (N = 34) | | Non-LD (N = 45) | |
|---|---|---|---|---|
| Scale | Mean | SD | Mean | SD |
| Aggression | 4.7 | 3.8 | 5.7 | 4.4 |
| Inhibition | 6.8 | 2.4 | 6.8 | 2.7 |
| Activity level | 5.6 | 2.4 | 5.6 | 2.3 |
| Sleep disturbance | 2.1 | 1.8 | 2.2 | 2.0 |
| Somatization | 1.8 | 1.5 | 2.5 | 1.5 |
| Sociability | 7.2 | 2.2 | 6.8 | 2.6 |

TABLE 11.  Frequency of MCBC Behavior Profiles Demonstrated by Learning Disabled and Non–Learning Disabled Children Seen in a Developmental Disabilities Center

| Profile | LD (N = 34) | Non-LD (N = 45) |
|---|---|---|
| Behavior Problem Profiles | 20 (59%) | 31 (69%) |
| Internalizing | 19 (56) | 24 (53) |
| Inhibited-Nonaggressive | 18 (53) | 20 (44) |
| Low Social Skills | 1 (3) | 4 (9) |
| Externalizing | 1 (3) | 7 (16) |
| Aggressive-Inhibited | 1 (3) | 3 (7) |
| Mildly Aggressive | 0 (0) | 0 (0) |
| Aggressive-Active | 0 (0) | 3 (7) |
| Undifferentiated | 0 (0) | 1 (2) |
| Behavior-Problem Free | 2 (6) | 3 (7) |
| Unclassified | 12 (35) | 11 (24) |

specific Behavior-Problem Profile there was also no significant difference in frequency of occurrence between the LD and non-LD groups. It can be seen that the most frequently demonstrated profile by both groups was the Inhibited-Nonaggressive profile (56 percent of the LD group and 53 percent of the non-LD group). Very few externalizing behavior problem profiles were demonstrated by either group (3 percent of the LD group and 16 percent of the non-LD group). In fact, of the total of Behavior-Problem profiles demonstrated, nineteen out of twenty or 95 percent for the LD group and twenty-four out of thirty-one or 77 percent for the non-LD group were of the internalizing type.

Thus, the results of this study provided no support for the notion that learning disabled children (classified as learning disabled on the basis of intellectual and academic performance) demonstrate more behavior problems or different types of behavior problems than children with poor school performance who were not classified as learning disabled.

To explore further this lack of differences in behavior problems among subgroups of children with poor school performance who were referred to a developmental disabilities clinic, additional subgroups were derived and the data was reanalyzed. It was decided to subdivide further the non-LD group on the basis of level of intellectual functioning. A mental retardation subgroup (MR) was delineated for those children with WISC-R Full-Scale IQ < 70. A borderline subgroup was formed consisting of children with WISC-R Full Scale IQ > 70 < 84. Finally, a residual subgroup was formed consisting of children not LD, MR, or Borderline.

Table 12 depicts the means and standard deviations for the various subgroups of children with poor school performance who were seen at the DEC. Overall one-way analysis of variance (ANOVA) was conducted for each MCBC scale. There were no significant differences among the subgroups on the Aggression, Activity Level, Sleep Disturbance, or Somatization scales. There was a significant difference on the Inhibition scale ($F = 3.23, p < .03$). Internal analysis using the Duncan Multiple Range Test revealed that the MR subgroup was significantly higher ($p < .09$) than the Residual and Borderline subgroups, with the other groups not differing significantly among themselves. There also was a significant difference on the Somatization scale (F $= 3.67, p < .02$), with internal analysis showing that the MR subgroup was significantly ($p < .05$) higher than the other subgroups, which did not differ significantly among themselves.

Table 13 presents the means and standard deviations for the intellectual and academic achievement test scores for the various subgroups of children with poor school performance who were seen at the DEC. Overall one-way ANOVA revealed highly significant differences ($p < .0001$) among the subgroups in terms of Verbal Scale IQ, Performance Scale IQ, Full Scale IQ, and reading, math, written language, and knowledge cluster-achievement percentiles. Internal analysis using the Duncan Multiple Range Test indicated significant differences ($p < .05$) in means for all subgroups for Verbal, Performance, and Full Scale IQ. The residual subgroup demonstrated the highest, followed by the LD, Borderline, and MR subgroups in each instance. In terms of achievement-test scores for reading and written language, the Residual subgroup was significantly higher than the other subgroups, which did not differ significantly among themselves. On math and knowledge scores, the LD and Borderline subgroups did not differ significantly from each other, but the Residual

TABLE 12. Mean and Standard Deviation of MCBC Scale Ratings for Subgroups of Developmentally Disabled Children

| Scale | LD (N = 34) Mean | SD | Mentally Retarded (N = 14) Mean | SD | Borderline (N = 14) Mean | SD | Residual (N = 17) Mean | SD |
|---|---|---|---|---|---|---|---|---|
| Aggression | 4.7 | 3.8 | 5.5 | 4.1 | 5.0 | 4.4 | 6.5 | 4.8 |
| Inhibition | 6.8 | 2.4 | 8.4 | 2.6 | 6.6 | 2.8 | 5.6 | 2.3 |
| Activity level | 5.6 | 2.4 | 6.0 | 2.7 | 4.7 | 2.5 | 6.0 | 1.5 |
| Sleep disturbance | 2.1 | 1.8 | 2.5 | 2.0 | 2.1 | 2.2 | 2.0 | 1.9 |
| Somatization | 1.8 | 1.5 | 3.4 | 1.6 | 1.9 | 1.4 | 2.2 | 1.2 |
| Sociability | 7.2 | 2.2 | 6.6 | 3.0 | 6.0 | 2.7 | 7.5 | 2.1 |

subgroup was significantly higher and the MR subgroup was significantly lower than all other subgroups.

Table 14 presents the frequency and percentage occurrence of MCBC behavior profiles demonstrated by the various subgroups of developmentally disabled children. In terms of category of behavior profiles, 59 percent of the LD, 64 percent of the MR, 64 percent of the Borderline, and 76 percent of the Residual subgroups demonstrated a behavior-problem profile. The Behavior-Problem-Free profile was demonstrated by 6 percent of the LD, 0 percent of the MR, 7 percent of the Borderline, and 12 percent of the Residual subgroups. The unclassified category represented 35 percent of the LD, 36 percent of the MR, 29 percent of the Borderline, and 12 percent of the Residual subgroups. There was no significant difference in the frequency of occurrence of these behavior profile categories across the various subgroups as reflected by chi square. In terms of each spe-

TABLE 13.   Mean and Standard Deviation of Intellectual and Achievement Test Scores for Subgroups of Developmentally Disabled Children

| Measure | LD (N = 34) | | Mentally Retarded (N = 14) | | Borderline (N = 14) | | Residual (N = 17) | |
|---|---|---|---|---|---|---|---|---|
| | Mean | SD | Mean | SD | Mean | SD | Mean | SD |
| WISC-R | | | | | | | | |
| Verbal Scale IQ | 85.8 | 12.0 | 65.9 | 7.8 | 77.9 | 7.2 | 107.6 | 10.2 |
| Performance Scale IQ | 90.5 | 9.8 | 64.4 | 9.2 | 74.9 | 7.1 | 104.9 | 10.4 |
| Full Scale IQ | 87.2 | 8.6 | 63.8 | 6.1 | 74.6 | 3.2 | 106.8 | 9.5 |
| Woodcock Johnson Psychoeducational Battery[a] | | | | | | | | |
| Reading cluster | 17.5 | 16.4 | 8.9 | 13.1 | 11.4 | 13.5 | 72.1 | 21.9 |
| Math cluster | 15.9 | 15.6 | 2.1 | 3.8 | 10.6 | 12.0 | 64.9 | 22.0 |
| Written language cluster | 15.9 | 16.9 | 8.9 | 12.0 | 15.0 | 19.8 | 66.9 | 19.4 |
| Knowledge cluster | 23.5 | 22.0 | 3.1 | 3.8 | 11.5 | 14.2 | 73.0 | 20.6 |

[a]Percentile scores for age

cific Behavior-Problem Profile, there was also no significant difference in frequency of occurrence among the subgroups of developmentally disabled children. The most frequently demonstrated Behavior-Problem Profile was the Inhibited-Nonagressive in 53 percent of the LD, 50 percent of the MR, 43 percent of the Borderline, and 41 percent of the Residual subgroups. Externalizing Behavior-Problem Profiles were very infrequent, being demonstrated by only 3 percent of the LD, 7 percent of the MR and of the Borderline subgroups, but 29 percent of the Residual subgroup. Of the total Behavior-Problem Profiles, internalizing types constituted 95 percent of those demonstrated by the LD subgroup, 89 percent of those demonstrated by the MR subgroup and by the Borderline subgroup, and 62 percent of those demonstrated by the Residual subgroup.

   One limitation of this study is the reliance upon intellectual and academic performance criteria for the classification of learning disability. There was no utilization of neurological dysfunction criteria. Thus, generalization of the findings needs to be appropriately limited. The primary purpose of the study was to investigate whether subgroups of children with poor school performance seen in a clinic for developmentally disabled children demonstrate differences in behavior problems. The findings indi-

TABLE 14.  Frequency of MCBC Behavior Profiles Demonstrated by Subgroups of Developmentally Disabled Children

| Profile | LD (N = 34) | Mentally Retarded (N = 14) | Borderline (N = 14) | Residual (N = 17) |
|---|---|---|---|---|
| Behavior Problem Profiles | 20 (59%) | 9 (64%) | 9 (64%) | 13 (76%) |
| Internalizing | 19 (56) | 8 (57) | 8 (57) | 8 (47) |
| Inhibited-Nonaggressive | 18 (53) | 7 (50) | 6 (43) | 7 (41) |
| Low Social Skills | 1 (3) | 1 (7) | 2 (14) | 1 (5) |
| Externalizing | 1 (3) | 1 (7) | 1 (7) | 5 (29) |
| Aggressive-Inhibited | 1 (3) | 1 (7) | 0 (0) | 2 (12) |
| Mildly Aggressive | 0 (0) | 0 (0) | 0 (0) | 0 (0) |
| Aggressive-Active | 0 (0) | 0 (0) | 1 (7) | 2 (12) |
| Undifferentiated | 0 (0) | 0 (0) | 0 (0) | 1 (6) |
| Behavior-Problem Free | 2 (6) | 0 (0) | 1 (7) | 2 (12) |
| Unclassified | 12 (35) | 5 (36) | 4 (29) | 2 (12) |

cate that these subgroups of developmentally disabled children differed significantly and meaningfully in terms of intellectual level of functioning and academic achievement functioning. However, there were no significant differences in behavior problems as reflected in MCBC scale scores or Behavior Profiles. As a total group, forty-three out of seventy-nine, or 54 percent, demonstrated an Internalizing Behavior-Problem Profile; eight out of seventy-nine, or 10 percent, an Externalizing Behavior-Problem Profile; five out of seventy-nine, or 6 percent, a Behavior-Problem-Free Profile; and twenty-three out of seventy-nine, or 29 percent, were unclassified. Thus, while not demonstrating differences in behavior problems as a function of subgroups, overall the most frequent behavior-problem profile was of an internalizing type. This is in contrast to the prominence of externalizing profiles that we have previously found to characterize children referred to psychiatric clinics. The fact that 29 percent of the residual group demonstrated an externalizing Behavior-Problem Profile suggests that perhaps the poor school performance of this subgroup was attributable to behavior problems.

CHAPTER 7

# Conclusion and
# Future Directions

It has been asserted that the study of behavior problems and learning disabilities has been hampered by the lack of an empirically based system for delineating and classifying behavior problems and by the reliance upon a main-effects etiological model that viewed learning and behavior problems as either organically or psychogenically based. However, progress is being made in delineating empirically based patterns of behavior problems and in utilizing interactional models that seek to evaluate the role of biological, psychological, and situational variables in behavior and learning disorders. The study of behavior problems in children who are confronted with the task of coping with chronic childhood illnesses and disorders is one interactional model that offers promise in terms of the clinical utility of the knowledge yielded.

Several main findings reflect our knowledge to date regarding behavior problems. There are many behavior problems demonstrated in childhood, but factor-analytic studies have shown that this array of behavior problems can be reduced to a number of narrow-band syndromes and the ubiquitous broad-band syndromes of externalizing-conduct problems and internalizing-personality problems, respectively. These dimensions have been identified in many populations of nonreferred and referred children, including those with learning problems as well as those with other developmental and clinical problems. The findings in general, and in terms of group differences, have been that: children referred for care exhibit behavior problems several times as severe or frequent as nonreferred children; those with developmental disabilities, and the subgroup with learning problems, demonstrate more behavioral disturbance than normals but less and different types than children referred for psychiatric care; and children with externalizing-conduct problems have poorer outcomes than those with internalizing-personality problems.

However, we have also learned that the frequency of behavior problems in the normal population is high and that there is some stability in behavior dimensions over time; but the consistency is generally insufficient, except in the situation of psychosis or antisocial behavior, to derive accurate prognostic statements for individuals. Even with children demonstrating highly antisocial behavior, only 50 percent demonstrate highly antisocial behavior as adults. Furthermore, while the correlations between multiple raters are reasonably high, the amount of agreement decreases considerably if the raters are rating behavior in different situations such as at home and at school.

Somewhat parallel to the line of empirical research on delineating behavior problems in children has been the use of peer nominations to gather information about the social relationships of children with learning and/or behavioral problems. This line of research has augmented our understanding of the correlates of behavior problems in terms of social relationships with peers and adults and ways of processing social information. There is ample support for the ability of peer nomination to identify groups of children that differ behaviorally and in their social relationships and in social-information processing. Again we see the delineation of aggressive and withdrawn subgroups with poorer outcome associated with aggression. The addition of social status or popularity dimensions and social processing dimensions makes possible the formation of subgroups on the basis of multidimensional classification. Such a multidimensional matrix offers the potential for increasing the accuracy of prognostic assessments as well as providing a basis for specificity of intervention along multiple dimensions simultaneously.

The advances in our understanding of behavior problems

have been reflected in a more considered view of the issue of behavior problems in children with learning disabilities. The field has progressed from a categorical model that viewed school maladjustment as either a learning problem or an emotional problem to a focus upon an underlying continuum of interacting personality and impairment factors. The increased capability for delineating behavior problems has provided information about the relative frequency of various types of internalizing and externalizing behavior problems in children with learning disabilities. The contention of a particular link of learning disabilities with one type of behavior problem—delinquency—is now tempered by evidence of increased frequencies of inhibited behavior problem patterns that are perhaps less noticeable. Such evidence also serves to stimulate conceptualization of the interaction of learning and behavioral problems to be less simplistic and more multidimensional.

The efforts to empirically delineate subgroups among the learning disabled is yielding interesting results. In addition to delineations on the basis of behavior, the dimensions of social relationships and patterns of neuropsychological functioning have also been utilized. Through such efforts the multidimensional matrix evolves in its ability to represent clinically meaningful dimensions of children's functioning.

However, the most compelling need now is for enhancement through theory. The methodology has outstripped the integration of the findings and formulation of relationships among the various components and parameters, particularly in terms of etiology and outcome.

Theorists need to be encouraged to join the empiricists in making sense out of the findings that are forthcoming and in directing future research endeavors. There is cause for encouragement. The inclusion of a focus on the role of mediating variables, both those in the situation and in the individual, provides a vehicle for enhancing our understanding of vulnerable and invulnerable children. One such mediating variable is the process of parent-child interaction at various points in the life-span. Our own line of research has expanded to incorporate a focus on another mediating variable: the role of cognitive processes in mediating stress associated with developmental, learning, and other chronic childhood illnesses and disorders. Although most studies still employ a main effects model, there is increasing recognition of the need to develop and utilize interactional models that seek to evaluate the role of biological, psychological, and situational variables in the etiology, prevention, and remediation of behavior disorders. The primary contention is that we will enhance the clinical utility of our empirical approaches to the extent that we can formulate and test hypotheses about the interrelationship of factors.

# References

Achenbach, T. M. 1966. "The Classification of Children's Psychiatric Symptoms: A Factor Analytic Study." *Psychological Monographs,* 80:7.

————. 1978. "The Child Behavior Profile: I. Boys Aged 6–11." *Journal of Consulting and Clinical Psychology* 46:478–88.

————. 1979. "The Child Behavior Profile: An Empirically Based System for Assessing Children's Behavioral Problems and Competencies." *International Journal of Mental Health* 7:24–42.

Achenbach, T. M., and Edelbrock, C. S. 1978. "The Classification of Child Psychopathology: A Review and Analysis of Empirical Effects." *Psychological Bulletin* 85:1275–1301.

————. 1979. "The Child Behavior Profile: II. Boys Aged 12–16 and Girls Aged 6–11 and 12–16." *Journal of Consulting and Clinical Psychology* 47:223–33.

————. 1981. "Behavioral Problems and Competencies Reported by Parents of Normal and Disturbed Children Aged 4–16." *Monographs of the Society for Research in Child Development* 46 (1): 1–82.

Achenbach, T. M., and Lewis, M. 1971. "A Proposed Model for Clinical Research and Its Application to Encopresis and Enuresis." *Journal of the American Academy of Child Psychiatry* 10:535–54.

Berman, A. 1972. "Neurological Dysfunction in Juvenile Delinquency: Implications for Early Intervention." *Child Care Quarterly* 1:264–71.

————. 1974. "Delinquents Are Disabled." In *Youth in Trouble,* edited by B. Kratoville. San Rafael, Calif.: Academic Press.

————. 1981. "Research Associating Learning Disabilities with Juvenile Delinquency." In *Developmental Theory and Research in Learning Disabilities,* edited by J. Gottlieb and S. S. Strichart, 244–77. Baltimore: University Park Press.

Berman, A. and Siegal, A. 1976a. "A Neurological Approach to the Etiology, Prevention and Treatment of Juvenile Delinquency." In *Child Personality and Psychopathology: Current Topics,* edited by A. Davids, vol. 3. New York: Wiley-Interscience.

————. 1976b. "A Neuropsychological Approach to Adaptive and

Learning Deficits in Delinquent Males." *Journal of Learning Disabilities* 9:583–90.

Broder, P. K.; Dunivant, N.; Smith, E. C.; and Sutton, L. P. 1981. "Further Observations on the Link between Learning Disabilities and Juvenile Delinquency." *Journal of Educational Psychology* 73: 838–50.

Bryan, J. H. 1981. "Social Behaviors of Learning Disabled Children." In *Developmental Theory and Research in Learning Disabilities,* edited by J. Gottlieb and S. S. Strichart, 215–43. Baltimore: University Park Press.

Bryan, T. H. 1974a. "An Observational Analysis of Classroom Behaviors of Children with Learning Disabilities." *Journal of Learning Disabilities* 7:26–34.

———. 1974b. "Peer Popularity of Learning Disabled Children." *Journal of Learning Disabilities* 7:621–25.

———. 1977. "Learning Disabled Children's Comprehension of Nonverbal Communication." *Journal of Learning Disabilities* 10:501–6.

———. 1978. "Social Relationships and Verbal Interactions of Learning Disabled Children." *Journal of Learning Disabilities* 11: 107–15.

Bryan, T. H. and Wheeler, R. 1972. "Perception of Children with Learning Disabilities: The Eye of the Observer." *Journal of Learning Disabilities* 5:484–88.

Campbell, S. B. 1974. "Cognitive Styles and Behavior Problems of Clinic Boys: A Comparison of Epileptic, Hyperactive, Learning Disabled, and Normal Groups." *Journal of Abnormal Child Psychology* 2: 307–12.

Clements, S., and Peters, J. 1962. "Minimal Brain Dysfunctions in the School-Age Child." *Archives of General Psychiatry* 6:185–97.

Coie, J. D.; Dodge, K. A.; and Cappotelli, H. 1982. "Dimensions and Types of Social Status: A Cross-Age Perspective." *Developmental Psychology* 18:557–70.

Coleman, J.; Wolkind, S.; and Ashley, L. 1977. "Symptoms of Behavior Disturbance and Adjustment to School." *Journal of Child Psychology and Psychiatry* 18:201–9.

Coleman, J. C. and Sandhu, M. 1967. "A Descriptive Relational Study of 364 Children Referred to a University Clinic for Learning Disorders." *Psychological Reports* 20:1091–1105.

Connolly, C. 1971. "Social and Emotional Factors in Learning Disabilities." In *Progress In Learning Disabilities,* edited by H. R. Myklebust, vol. 2. New York: Grune and Stratton, Inc.

Crowther, J. H.; Bond, L. A.; and Rolf, J. C. 1981. "The Incidence, Prevalence, and Severity of Behavior Disorders among Preschool-

Aged Children in Day Care." *Journal of Abnormal Child Psychology* 9:23–42.

Cullinan, D.; Epstein, M. H.; and Dembinski, R. J. 1979. "Behavior Problems of Educationally Handicapped and Normal Pupils." *Journal of Abnormal Child Psychology* 7:495–502.

Curry, J. F., and Thompson, R. J., Jr. 1979. "The Utility of Behavior Checklist Ratings in Differentiating Developmentally Disabled from Psychiatrically Referred Children." *Journal of Pediatric Psychology* 4:345–52.

———. 1982. "Patterns of Behavioral Disturbance in Developmentally Disabled Children: A Replicated Cluster Analysis." *Journal of Pediatric Psychology* 7:61–73.

———. 1985. "Patterns of Behavioral Disturbance in Developmentally Disabled and Psychiatrically Referred Children: A Cluster Analytic Approach." *Journal of Pediatric Psychology* 10:151–67.

Defilippis, N. A. 1979. "Normative and Validity Data for the Missouri Children's Behavior Checklist." *Journal of Clinical Psychology* 35: 605–10.

Delamater, A. M., and Lahey, B. B. 1983. "Physiological Correlates of Conduct Problems and Anxiety in Hyperactive and Learning Disabled Children." *Journal of Abnormal Child Psychology* 11:85–100.

Delamater, A. M.; Lahey, B. B.; and Drake, L. 1981. "Toward an Empirical Subclassification of 'Learning Disabilities'. A Psychophysical Comparison of 'Hyperactive' and 'Nonhyperactive' Subgroups." *Journal of Abnormal Child Psychology* 9:65–77.

Dodge, K. A. (1985). "Attributional Bias in Aggressive Children." In *Advances in Cognitive-Behavioral Research and Therapy,* edited by P. Kendall, vol. 4. New York: Academic Press.

Dodge, K. A.; Coie, J. D.; and Brakke, N. P. 1982. "Behavior Patterns of Socially Rejected and Neglected Preadolescents: The Roles of Social Approach and Aggression." *Journal of Abnormal Child Psychology* 10:389–410.

Dreger, R. M. 1981. "First, Second, and Third-Order Factors from the Children's Behavioral Classification Project Instrument and an Attempt at Rapprochement." *Journal of Abnormal Psychology* 90: 242–60.

Edelbrock, C., and Achenbach, T. M. 1980. "A Typology of Child Behavior Profile Patterns." *Journal of Abnormal Child Psychology* 8:441–70.

Evans, W. R. 1975. "The Behavior Problem Checklist: Data from an Inner-City Population." *Psychology in the Schools* 12:301–3.

Everitt, B. 1980. *Cluster Analysis,* 2d ed. New York: Halsted Press.

Forness, S. R.; Rubano, R.; Rotberg, J.; Bender, M.; Gardner, T.; Lynch,

E.; and Zemanek, D. 1980. "Identifying Children with School Learning and Behavior Problems Served by Interdisciplinary Clinics and Hospitals." *Child Psychiatry and Human Development* 11:67-78.

Gajar, A. 1979. "Educable Mentally Retarded, Learning Disabled, Emotionally Disturbed: Similarities and Differences." *Exceptional Children* 45:470-72.

Gersten, J. C.; Langner, T. S.; Eisenberg, J. B.; Simcha-Fagen, O.; and McCarthy, E. D. 1976. "Stability and Change in Types of Behavioral Disturbance of Children and Adolescents." *Journal of Abnormal Child Psychology* 4:111-27.

Gersten, J. C.; Langner, T. S.; and Simcha-Fagen, O. 1979. "Development Patterns of Types of Behavioral Disturbance and Secondary Prevention." *International Journal of Mental Health* 7:132-49.

Grieger, R. M., and Richards, H. C. 1976. "Prevalence and Structure of Behavior Symptoms among Children in Special Education and Regular Classroom Settings." *Journal of School Psychology* 14:27-38.

Jampolsky, G. G. 1965. "Psychiatric Considerations in Reading Disorders." In *Reading Disorders*, edited by R. M. Flower, H. F. Grofman, and L. I. Lawson. Philadelphia: Davis Co.

Jenkins, S.; Bax, M.; and Hart, H. 1980. "Behavior Problems in Pre-School Children." *Journal of Child Psychology and Psychiatry and Allied Disciplines* 21:5-17.

Johnson, S. C. 1967. "Hierarchical Clustering Schemes." *Psychometrika* 32:241-54.

Kenny, T. J., and Clemmens, R. L. 1971. "Medical and Psychological Correlates in Children with Learning Disabilities." *Journal of Pediatrics* 78:273-77.

Klein, E. 1949. "Psychoanalytic Aspects of School Problems." *Psychoanalytic Study of the Child* 3:369-90.

Kohlberg, L.; LaCross, J.; and Rick, D. 1972. "The Predictability of Adult Mental Health from Childhood Behavior." In *Manual of Child Psychopathology* edited by B. B. Wolman. New York: McGraw-Hill.

Kohn, M. 1977. *School Competence, Symptoms, and Underachievement in Childhood: A Longitudinal Perspective.* Washington, D. C.: Winston Wiley.

Kohn, M., and Rosman, B. 1972a. "A Social Competence Scale and Symptom Checklist for the Preschool Child: Factor Dimensions, Their Cross-Instrument Generality and Longitudinal Persistence." *Developmental Psychology* 6:430-44.

———. 1972b. "Relationship of Preschool Social-Emotional Functioning to Later Intellectual Achievement." *Developmental Psychology* 6:445-52.

Lahey, B. B.; Stempniak, M.; Robinson, E., Jr.; and Tyroler, M. J. 1978.

"Hyperactivity and Learning Disabilities as Independent Dimensions of Child Behavior Problems." *Journal of Abnormal Psychology* 87: 333–40.

Lane, B. A. 1980. "The Relationship of Learning Disabilities to Juvenile Delinquency: Current Status." *Journal of Learning Disabilities* 13: 425–34.

Langhorne, J. E., Jr., and Loney, J. 1979. "A Fourfold Model for Sub-grouping the Hyperkinetic/MBD Syndrome." *Child Psychiatry and Human Development* 9:153–59.

Langhorne, J. E., Jr.; Loney, J.; Paternite, C. E.; and Bechtoldt, H. P. 1976. "Childhood Hyperkinesis: A Return to the Source." *Journal of Abnormal Psychology* 85:201–9.

Larrivee, B., and Bourque, M. L. 1981. "Factor Structure of Classroom Behavior Problems for Mainstreamed and Regular Students." *Journal of Abnormal Child Psychology* 9:399–406.

Ledingham, J. E. 1981. "Developmental Patterns of Aggressive and Withdrawn Behavior in Childhood: A Possible Method for Identifying Preschizophrenics." *Journal of Abnormal Child Psychology* 9: 1–22.

Ledingham, J. E., and Schwartzman, A. E. 1984. "A Three-Year Follow-Up of Aggressive and Withdrawn Behavior in Childhood: Preliminary Findings." *Journal of Abnormal Child Psychology* 12: 157–68.

Leong, C. K. 1982. "Promising Areas of Research into Learning Disabilities with Emphasis on Reading Disabilities." In *Theory and Research in Learning Disabilities,* edited by J. P. Das, R. F. Mulcahy, and A. E. Wall. New York: Plenum Press.

Levitt, E. E. 1957. "The Results of Psychotherapy with Children: An Evaluation." *Journal of Consulting Psychology* 21:186–89.

———. 1971. "Research on Psychotherapy with Children." In *Handbook of Psychotherapy and Behavior Change,* edited by A. E. Bergin and S. Garfield. New York: John Wiley and Sons.

Levy, H. 1973. *Square Pegs in Round Holes.* Boston: Little, Brown.

Lindholm, B. W., and Touliatos, J. 1976. "Comparison of Children in Regular and Special Education Classes on the Behavior Problem Checklist." *Psychological Reports* 38:451–58.

Lindholm, B. W., and Touliatos, J. 1981. "Development of Children's Behavior Problems." *The Journal of Genetic Psychology* 139:47–53.

Loney, J.; Kramer, J.; and Milich, R. 1981. "The Hyperkinetic Child Grows Up: Predictors of Symptom, Delinquency, and Achievement at Follow-Up." In *Psychosocial Aspects of Drug Treatment for Hyperactivity* edited by K. Gadow and J. Loney. Boulder, Col.: Westview Press.

Loney, J.; Langhorne, J. E., Jr.; and Paternite, C. E. 1978. "An Empirical Basis for Subgrouping the Hyperkinetic/Minimal Brain Dysfunction Syndrome." *Journal of Abnormal Psychology* 87:431-41.

Mattsson, A. 1972. "Long-Term Physical Illness in Childhood: A Challenge to Psychosocial Adaptation." *Pediatrics* 50:801-11.

McCarthy, J. M., and Paraskevopoulos, J. 1969. "Behavior Patterns of Learning Disabled, Emotionally Disturbed, and Average Children." *Exceptional Children* 36:69-74.

McDermott, P. A. 1980. "Prevalence and Consistency of Behavioral Disturbance Taxonomies in the Regular School Population." *Journal of Abnormal Child Psychology* 8:523-36.

McKinney, J. D. 1984. "The Search for Subtypes of Specific Learning Disability." *Journal of Learning Disabilities* 17:43-50.

Milich, R., and Dodge, K. A. 1984. "Social Information Processing in Child Psychiatric Populations." *Journal of Abnormal Child Psychology* 12:471-90.

Milich, R., and Landau, S. 1984. "A Comparison of the Social Status and Social Behavior of Aggressive and Aggressive/Withdrawn Boys." *Journal of Abnormal Child Psychology* 12:277-88.

Murray, C. 1976. *The Link Between Learning Disabilities and Juvenile Delinquency.* Washington, D.C.: American Institute for Research.

O'Donnell, J. P., and Van Tuinan, M. 1979. "Behavior Problems of Preschool Children: Dimensions and Congenital Correlates." *Journal of Abnormal Child Psychology* 7:61-75.

Pearson, G. H. 1955. "A Survey of Learning Difficulties in Young Children." *The Psychoanalytic Study of the Child.* New York: International University Press.

Pekarik, E. G.; Prinz, R. J.; Liebert, D. E.; Weintraub, S.; and Neale, J. M. 1976. "The Pupil Evaluation Inventory: A Sociometric Technique for Assessing Children's Social Behavior." *Journal of Abnormal Child Psychology* 4:83-97.

Peterson, D. R. 1961. "Behavior Problems of Middle Childhood." *Journal of Consulting Psychology* 25:205-9.

Pless, I. B., and Douglas, J. W. B. 1971. "Chronic Illness in Childhood: Part I. Epidemiological and Clinical Characteristics." *Pediatrics* 47: 405-14.

Pless, I. B., and Pinkerton, P. 1975. *Chronic Childhood Disorders: Promoting Patterns of Adjustment.* London: Kempton.

Pless, I. B., and Roghmann, K. J. 1971. "Chronic Illness and its Consequences: Observations Based on Three Epidemiologic Surveys." *Journal of Pediatrics* 79:351-59.

Pless, I. B.; Roghmann, K.; and Haggerty, R. J. 1972. "Chronic Illness, Family Functioning, and Psychological Adjustment: A Model for the

Allocation of Preventive Mental Health Services." *International Journal of Epidemiology* 1:271–77.

Pless, I. B., and Satterwhite, B. B. 1975. "Chronic Illness." In *Child Health and the Community,* edited by R. Haggerty, K. Roghmann, and I. Pless. New York: John Wiley and Sons.

Quay, H. 1977. "Measuring Dimensions of Deviant Behavior: The Behavior Problem Checklist." *Journal of Abnormal Child Psychology* 5:277–87.

———. 1983. "A Dimensional Approach to Behavior Disorder: The Revised Behavior Problem Checklist." *School Psychology Review* 12:244–49.

Quay, H. C., and Gredler, Y. 1981. "Dimensions of Problem Behavior in Institutionalized Retardates." *Journal of Abnormal Child Psychology* 9:523–28.

Quay, H. C., and Peterson, D. R. 1967. *Manual for the Behavior Problem Checklist.* Champaign, Ill.: Children's Research Center, University of Illinois.

Richardson, S.; Brutlen, M.; and Nagel, C. 1973. *Something's Wrong with My Child.* New York: Harcourt Brace Jovanovich.

Richman, M.; Stevenson, J.; and Graham, P. 1975. "Prevalence of Behavior Problems in Three-Year-Old Children: An Epidemiological Study in a London Borough." *Journal of Child Psychology and Psychiatry* 16:277–87.

Robbins, D. M.; Beck, J. C.; Prier, R.; Cags, D.; Jacobs, D.; and Smith, C. 1983. "Learning Disability and Neuropsychological Impairment in Adjudicated Unincarcerated Male Delinquents." *Journal of the American Academy of Child Psychiatry* 22:40–46.

Robins, L. N. 1966. *Deviant Children Grow Up.* Baltimore: Williams and Wilkins.

———. 1978. "Sturdy Childhood Predictors of Adult Antisocial Behaviour: Replications from Longitudinal Studies." *Psychological Medicine* 8:611–22.

———. 1979. "Follow-Up Studies." In *Psychopathological Disorders of Childhood.* 2d ed., edited by H. C. Quay and J. S. Werry. New York: John Wiley and Sons.

Roff, M. 1972. "A Two-Factor Approach to Juvenile Delinquency and the Later Histories of Juvenile Delinquents." In *Life History Research in Psychopathology,* edited by M. Roff, L. N. Robins, and M. Plollack, vol. 2, pp. 77–101. Minneapolis: University of Minnesota Press.

Roff, J. D., and Wirt, R. D. 1984. "Childhood Aggression and Social Adjustment as Antecedents of Delinquency." *Journal of Abnormal Child Psychology* 12:111–26.

Rosenthal, R.; Hall, J. A.; Archer, D.; DiMatteo, M. R.; and Rogers, P. L. 1977. "The PONS Test: Measuring Sensitivity to Nonverbal Cues." In *Advances in Psychological Assessment,* edited by P. McReynolds, vol. 4, pp. 179–221. San Francisco: Jossey-Bass.

Rosenthal, R.; Hall, J. A.; DiMatteo, M. R.; Rogers, P. L.; and Archer, D. 1979. *Sensitivity to Nonverbal Communication: The PONS Test.* Baltimore: Johns Hopkins University Press.

Rubin, E. Z. 1971. "Cognitive Dysfunction and Emotional Disorders." In *Progress in Learning Disabilities,* edited by H. R. Myklebust, vol. 2. New York: Grune and Stratton.

Satz, P., and Morris, R. 1981. "Learning Disability Subtypes: A Review." In *Neuropsychological and Cognitive Processes in Reading,* edited by F. J. Perozzolo and M. C. Wittrock. New York: Academic Press.

Schaefer, E. S. 1981. "Development of Adaptive Behavior: Conceptual Models and Family Correlates." In *Prevention of Retarded Development in Psychosocially Disadvantaged Children,* edited by M. Begab, H. Garber, and H. C. Haywood. Baltimore: University Park Press.

Sines, J. O.; Pauker, J. D.; Sines, L. K.; and Owen, D. R. 1969. "Identification of Clinically Relevant Dimensions of Children's Behavior." *Journal of Consulting and Clinical Psychology* 33:728–34.

Smith, L. 1976. *Improving Your Child's Behavior Chemistry.* New York: Simon and Schuster.

Speer, D. C. 1971. "The Behavior Problem Checklist: Baseline Data from Parents of Child Guidance and Nonclinic Children." *Journal of Consulting and Clinical Psychology* 36:221–28.

Spivack, G., and Spotts, J. 1966. *The Devereaux Child Behavior Rating Scale Manual.* Devon, Penn.: Devereaux Foundation.

Spivack, G., and Swift, M. 1967. *Devereaux Elementary School Behavior Rating Scale Manual.* Devon, Penn.: Devereaux Foundation Press.

Spreen, O. 1981. "The Relationship between Learning Disability, Neurological Impairment, and Delinquency: Results of a Follow-Up Study." *Journal of Nervous and Mental Disease* 169:791–99.

Stone, F. B. 1981. "Behavior Problems of Elementary-School Children." *Journal of Abnormal Child Psychology* 9:407–18.

Stone, W. L., and LaGreca, A. M. 1984. "Comprehension of Nonverbal Communication: A Reexamination of Social Competencies of Learning Disabled Children." *Journal of Abnormal Child Psychology* 12: 505–18.

Sylvester, E., and Kunst, M. 1943. "Psychodynamic Aspects of Reading Problems." *American Journal of Orthopsychiatry* 13:69–76.

Tavormina, J. B. 1975. "Relative Effectiveness of Behavioral and Reflective Group Counseling with Parents of Mentally Retarded Children." *Journal of Consulting and Clinical Psychology* 43:22–31.

Thompson, R. J., Jr. 1981. "Enhancing Coping with the Stress of Chronic Childhood Illness: A Heuristic Review." JSAS *Catalog of Selected Documents in Psychology* 11:(Ms. No. 2298).

———. 1982a. "Developmental Disabilities." In *Assessment Strategies in Behavioral Medicine*, edited by F. J. Keefe and J. A. Blumenthal. New York: Grune and Stratton.

———. 1982b. "Multidimensional Problems and Findings in Developmentally Disabled Children." *Journal of Developmental and Behavioral Pediatrics* 3:153–58.

———. 1984. "Behavior Problems in Developmentally Disabled Children." In *Advances in Developmental and Behavioral Pediatrics*, edited by D. K. Routh and M. L. Wolraich, vol. 5. Greenwich, Conn.: JAI Press.

———. 1985. "Coping with the Stress of Chronic Childhood Illness." In *Management of Chronic Disorders in Childhood*, edited by A. N. O'Quinn. Boston: G. K. Hall.

Thompson, R. J., Jr., and Curry, J. F. 1983. "A Construct Validity Study of the Missouri Children's Behavior Checklist with Developmentally Disabled Children." *Journal of Clinical Psychology* 39:691–95.

———. 1985. "Missouri Children's Behavior Checklist Profiles with Developmentally Disabled Children: Construct Validity." *Journal of Clinical Psychology* 41:556–64.

Thompson, R. J., Jr.; Curry, J. F.; Sturner, R. A.; Green, J. A.; and Funk, S. G. 1982. "Missouri Children's Behavior Checklist Ratings of Preschool Children as a Function of Risk Status for Developmental and Learning Problems." *Journal of Pediatric Psychology* 7:307–16.

Thompson, R. J., Jr.; Curry, J. F.; and Yancy, W. S. 1979. "The Utility of Parent's Behavior Checklist Ratings with Developmentally Disabled Children." *Journal of Pediatric Psychology* 4:19–28.

Thompson, R. J., Jr., and McAdoo, W. G. 1973. "A Comparison of Mothers' and Fathers' Behavior Checklist Ratings of Outpatient Boys and Girls." *Journal of Community Psychology* 1:387–89.

Thompson, R. J., Jr., and O'Quinn, A. N. 1979. *Developmental Disabilities: Etiologies, Manifestations, Diagnoses and Treatments.* New York: Oxford University Press.

Touliatos, J., and Lindholm, B. 1980. "Dimensions of Problem Behavior in Learning Disabled and Normal Children." *Perceptual and Motor Skills* 50:145–46.

Victor, J. B., and Halverson, C. F., Jr. 1976. "Behavior Problems in Elementary School Children: A Follow-Up Study." *Journal of Abnormal Child Psychology* 4:17–39.

Werry, J. S., and Quay, H. C. 1971. "The Prevalence of Behavior Symptoms in Younger Elementary School Children." *American Journal of Orthopsychiatry* 41:136–43.

Weintraub, S. A. 1973. "Self-Control as a Correlate of an Internalizing-Externalizing Symptom Dimension." *Journal of Abnormal Child Psychology* 1:292–307.

Wortes, J., and Wortes, H. 1968. "Who Comes to a Retardation Clinic: Implications for Social Planning." *American Journal of Public Health* 58:1746–52.

Zold, A. C., and Speer, D. C. 1971. "Follow-Up Study of Child Guidance Patients by Means of the Behavior Problem Checklist." *Journal of Clinical Psychology* 27:519–24.

# Index

## International Academy for Research In Learning Disabilities Monograph Series

Syracuse University Press

*A System of Marker Variables for the Field of Learning Disabilities*
Barbara K. Keogh et al.

The University of Michigan Press

*Rhyme and Reason in Reading and Spelling*
Lynette Bradley and Peter Bryant

*Drugs in Pregnancy and Childbirth: Infant Exposure and Maternal Information*
Yvonne Brackbill, Karen McManus, and Lynn Woodward

*Behavior Problems in Children with Developmental and Learning Disabilities*
Robert J. Thompson, Jr.